REINVENTING
THE PATIENT
EXPERIENCE

Strategies for Hospital Leaders

REINVENTING THE PATIENT EXPERIENCE

Strategies for Hospital Leaders

Jon B. Christianson, Ph.D.

Michael D. Finch, Ph.D.

Barbara Findlay, R.N., B.S.N.

Wayne B. Jonas, M.D.

Christine Goertz Choate, D.C., Ph.D.

ACHE Management Series

Health Administration Press

Your board, staff, or clients may also benefit from this book's insight. For more information on quantity discounts, contact the Health Administration Press Marketing Manager at (312) 424-9470.

Library of Congress Cataloging-in-Publication Data

Reinventing the patient experience : strategies for hospital leaders / Jon B. Christianson ... [et al.].
   p. cm.
   Includes bibliographical references.
   ISBN-13: 978-1-56793-278-2
   ISBN-10: 1-56793-278-2 (alk. paper)
1. Hospital care—United States. 2. Hospital patients—Care—United States. 3. Hospitals—United States—Administration. I. Christianson, Jon B. [DNLM: 1. Hospital-Patient Relations—United States. 2. Hospital Administration—methods—United States. WX 158.5 R374 2007]

RA965.6.R48 2007
362.11—dc22   2007012209

The paper used in this publication meets the minimum requirements of American National Standard for Information Sciences—Permanence of Paper for Printed Library Materials, ANSI Z39.48-1984.♾™

Acquisitions editor: Janet Davis; Project manager: Gregory Sebben; Layout editor and cover designer: Chris Underdown

Health Administration Press
A division of the Foundation of the
   American College of Healthcare Executives
1 North Franklin Street, Suite 1700
Chicago, IL 60606-3529
(312) 424-2800

Contents

Preface

A friend or family member is in the hospital, and you decide to visit. Your very first impression is disquieting. As you enter the hospital, the environment seems confusing and slightly intimidating, hardly welcoming. As you make your way to your friend's room—and it's not easy to find—you notice that the people you see, including the nurses, appear very intent on their work. But they don't seem very happy. They cluster in groups at the nurses' station, scrutinizing charts and filling out forms. No one looks up or acknowledges your presence as you search for your friend.

You find the right room, and your friend greets you with delight. She is surrounded by a tangle of equipment, and there is very little space for visitors, but you squeeze in. There is a window to the right of her bed; the view is of a brick wall of the adjoining hospital wing. After the usual small talk and exchange of stories about relatives and acquaintances, you ask if there is anything that you can do to make her more comfortable. You clear away her lunch, which, she notes, was delivered while she was out getting an MRI, was cold when she returned, and had been next to her bed for two hours. She is nauseated by the smell of the food but has been told by a passing nurse that someone would be there "soon" to remove it. While you are talking, a nurse enters the room and checks various readings on the equipment, changes something, and, with a distracted smile, moves quickly to the next room. You roll the food stand into the hallway and leave it there.

There is a steady stream of activity in the hallway, generating a significant amount of noise. This is punctuated periodically by overhead pages that sound slightly ominous to you and that are, at the least, disconcerting. Your friend observes that she has been having trouble sleeping because of the noise and mentions that a nurse has offered a pill to "help her get some rest." She declined the medication but wonders if she shouldn't reconsider.

At one point, a person in a white uniform enters the room, explaining to your friend that it is time for her walk. Your friend blanches at the suggestion, recounting that someone (who didn't explain who he was) had visited the room in the morning and told her to "take it easy" today. The staff person seems confused, spends a couple of minutes scrutinizing her chart, and leaves without comment. You then help your friend use the bathroom in her room, for which she is very appreciative. She was told to request help in getting out of bed to use the bathroom, but when she did so earlier that day, no one responded. She was able to manage on her own, although she caught her foot in some cables and almost fell. She wonders how she will do that night, when it's harder for her to see where to walk.

You ask your friend when she expects to be discharged and offer to drive her home. She isn't certain. She knows there has been some talk about discharge, but the resident has to reexamine her first. The last time that happened, six people packed into her room, talked with each other for some time about her "condition," and then left saying they would likely be back "later." No one has told her when that might be.

You promise to return the next day, bringing some "decent" coffee and her favorite dessert. As you are adjusting the channel on the television, your friend asks if you would check with the nurses about an inquiry she had made when admitted to the hospital. Apparently, she had received some relief from her pain through acupuncture treatments prior to her hospitalization and was hoping the acupuncturist could continue treating her while she was in the hospital. On your way out, you stop at the nurses' station to inquire about the status of your friend's request. The nurse says she hadn't heard about the request but promises to leave a note for the supervisor on the next shift.

As you make your way to the parking lot, you can't help but feel depressed by the visit. While your friend expects to fully recover and to return to her home soon, and the hospital apparently has the latest in technology (or at least its newsletter in the lobby suggests that's the case), you wonder if your friend is receiving the best possible care. Couldn't the environment be more conducive to healing? Couldn't the staff be more focused on patient care and, for that matter, your friend as a person? Why does your friend have to work so hard to get the attention of the hospital staff? Is it really necessary for her to be so anxious about her environment? Uncertain about what is happening? You decide that it would be a good idea to return earlier in the morning tomorrow—your friend could use the support.

We believe most readers of this book will relate readily to this narrative, or at least to parts of it, through their personal experiences. Technology has become a focal point for patient care in hospitals, and there is no disputing that it plays a major and essential role in modern medicine. Financial issues consume a significant portion of any hospital administrator's day, and there is no doubt that hospitals need to pay close attention to the bottom line to ensure that resources are adequate to provide the best care for their patients. Addressing staffing shortages seems to be a continuing problem for many hospitals, as does the need to respond to market pressures to control costs and improve patient safety. Relations between hospital administration and medical staff are strained as never before, with ongoing battles over where lucrative specialty services will be provided—in the hospital or in an outpatient facility owned by physicians. In this environment, it would seem easy enough for hospitals to be distracted from their focus on the patient experience. Yet some hospitals appear able to combine "high touch" with "high tech" care in an effective way. What can we learn from their experience that has value for the healthcare field and, ultimately, for the patients they serve?

This is the challenge that motivates this book. To address it, we have analyzed the experiences of eight highly diverse hospitals that all came to realize that they needed to transform the hospital experience for patients and their families in fundamental ways. They began with different resources at their disposal and faced different competitive pressures, but they were all sustained by a firm belief that it was "the right thing to do" for their patients.

Chapters 2 through 9 describe the experiences of each of the hospitals in implementing their strategies. These chapters, which are essentially eight case studies, are organized using a common structure. The first part of each chapter presents an executive summary of the hospital's experience. The rest of the chapter expands on this summary and provides greater detail, particularly around implementation issues. Each chapter contains brief perspectives of hospital leaders regarding particular aspects of their hospital's strategy and ends with a discussion of key success factors. Following these hospital-specific case studies, Chapters 10 and 11 recount important points made in a roundtable conversation involving representatives from seven of the eight hospitals. Chapter 10 focuses on implementation and operational issues relating to four areas: physical environment, nursing services, complementary therapies, and spirituality. In Chapter 11, the conversation shifts to issues of leadership and sustainability. In Chapter 12, we summarize cross-cutting findings from the hospital's experiences in implementing multifaceted strategies intended to reinvent the patient experience and discuss their implications for the healthcare field over the coming decade.

Jon B. Christianson, Ph.D.
Michael D. Finch, Ph.D.
Barbara Findlay, R.N., B.S.N.
Wayne B. Jonas, M.D.
Christine Goertz Choate, D.C., Ph.D.

Acknowledgments

This book would not have been possible to write without the willing participation of the eight hospitals we studied. The authors would like to thank Windber Medical Center (PA), St. Rose Dominican Hospitals–Siena Campus (NV), Abbott Northwestern Hospital (MN), Florida Hospital–Celebration Health (FL), Highline Medical Center (WA), St. Charles Medical Center–Bend (OR), North Hawaii Community Hospital (HI), The Valley Hospital (NJ), and especially all of the interviewees who carved space out of busy schedules to share their "found wisdom" with us. We would also like to acknowledge their capable support staff, who provided access to calendars, arranged meeting space and tours, and facilitated ongoing communication throughout the project. Our thanks as well go to those colleagues, research partners, and other formal and informal advisers who helped us identify and recruit the eight study hospitals.

We are grateful to Linda Cuoco, Lori Knutson, Nick Jacobs, Rich Keenan, Sid Mallory, Todd Sprague, Earl Bakken, Kathy Mitchell, Mark Benedum, Grace Henley, Paul Tucker, Ray Friel, Sally Grady, Stan Berry, and Vicky VanMeetren for permitting us to capture their expert knowledge and contagious enthusiasm in the direct quotes located throughout the book. Many of these same individuals generously participated in a day-long, face-to-face meeting in August 2006 to collectively analyze the study findings with us, confirm or challenge the themes we identified, and provide additional insight into their personal leadership strategies.

Sherry Loveless from the Samueli Institute Optimal Healing Environments Program provided tremendous administrative support for all aspects of this project, for which we are very appreciative. And finally, we thank the Samueli Institute for funding both the research reported in this book and the writing project itself.

CHAPTER 1

The Challenge to Hospitals: Reinventing the Patient Experience

The past decade has been tumultuous for hospitals. The industry has been "buffeted by conflicting forces," including "persistent over-capacity, misallocation of institutional assets and resources, low payment rates, aggressive competition from physician-owned entities and specialty hospitals and the increasing burden of uncompensated care."[1] For many hospitals, the focus has been on organizational survival. They have merged or affiliated with systems,[2] invested scarce resources in service expansions promising the greatest immediate returns,[3] and worked with medical staff physicians to reduce length of stay. For the industry as a whole, improvements have been made in financial measures.[4] But a recent American Hospital Association (AHA) report suggests that this focus on financial performance, along with a growing public perception that hospitals are error-prone environments, may be weakening public trust in hospitals as community institutions.[5]

Recent public opinion polls report that 56 percent of respondents trusted hospitals "some," "not much," or "not at all" to do the right thing.[6] In the late 1990s, the AHA launched an effort to track public perceptions of hospitals, and this effort has been continued by some state associations. The results suggest that a substantial portion of the public believes hospitals are "lacking individual identity, values and mission," having been "transformed from charitable institutions to purely business enterprises," and, as a result, are "impersonal and detached from community."[7] They put "economics ahead of patient care" and have abandoned their "traditional role as advocates for patient needs."[8] In sum, these survey findings suggest that many hospitals have lost the trust of the communities they serve.

This news could not come at a worse time for American hospitals, because consumers are becoming better informed about hospital performance and financially motivated to act on that information.[9] First-dollar health insurance coverage for hospital care is giving way to insurance products that feature higher deductibles and coinsurance rates, sometimes augmented by health savings accounts.[10] "Tiered network" products, although not yet common, contain financial incentives that reward patients who choose to obtain treatment at hospitals that score well on quality, cost, and patient satisfaction metrics.[11] Pay-for-performance programs reward hospitals directly for achieving benchmarks or performance improvements.[12] Comparative information on hospital performance is becoming more accessible to consumers on the Internet or through pamphlets and brochures provided by employers and health plans.[13] There is a presumption that these changes will influence consumers in their choice of hospitals. Although this remains an ongoing topic of debate and research, many hospitals are now engaged in programs to improve their patient satisfaction scores[14] and have increased their direct marketing to consumers.

The emerging era of consumerism in healthcare will force hospitals to reexamine their traditional organizational models and, in many cases, their cultures. In this book, we draw lessons from the experiences of a small group of hospitals that have been early innovators in implementing multidimensional strategies to reinvent the patient experience. What steps have they taken to pursue this goal? What roadblocks have they encountered? How have they overcome barriers? What have been the keys to their success? How does their experience translate to other hospitals? These are the questions we address in this book.

WHAT ARE THE COMPONENTS OF A REINVENTED PATIENT EXPERIENCE?

Rather than focusing on specific, targeted programs, we sought to identify hospitals that had developed broad yet integrated strategies for reinventing the patient experience. By doing so, we hoped to avoid the hospital "fad of the month" and to identify strategies that embodied deeper, presumably longer-lasting, organizational change.

In our environmental scan, we reviewed the hospital trade literature, participated in conferences and meetings where hospital innovators described their efforts, and sought out organizations that supported innovation in inpatient care. We concluded that a significant number of hospitals in the United States (we estimate between 200 and 400) were pursuing broad-based, multifaceted strategies to reinvent the patient experience. These hospitals had concluded that conventional training programs intended to make staff more "consumer friendly" were not sufficient by themselves to accomplish a fundamental change in the patient experience. And they reached this conclusion before the new consumerism in healthcare took center stage.

These hospitals did not employ a common language in describing why they embarked on their ambitious strategies. What was their motivation? Some hospital leaders cited a desire to create a "healing environment" within their hospital, while others talked about pursuing a "mind/body/spirit" approach to the care of hospitalized patients. Perhaps just as revealing is what these leaders did not speak of when justifying their efforts. They did not cite favorable financial projections or marketing considerations. Instead, they used phrases such as "It's the right thing to do," "It's what our patients want," and "It's the experience we would want for our family members or friends if they were hospitalized."

We found that hospitals typically drew from four different, but potentially mutually reinforcing, perspectives to develop a multifaceted strategy to reinvent the patient experience. One of these perspectives relates to environmental design.[15] The presumption is that the physical environment can influence not only the quality of the patient and family experience in the hospital but also the healing process itself. The literature provides numerous examples of facilities designed to minimize stress (e.g., through the use of water features, soundproofing, and artwork), support family involvement (e.g., through larger rooms, convenient family spaces, and kitchens), and remove physical barriers between nurses and patients.[16]

A second perspective concerns how nursing services should be provided in the hospital. Where this was an important component of hospital strategies, the hospital leaders emphasized a more "personalized" relationship between nurses and patients, with more "hands-on" care provided by nurses at the bedside. The goal is to reduce patient anxiety, improve communication regarding the patient's condition, and promote healing.[17] This approach to hospital nursing certainly is not new—in fact, it has a "back to the future" feeling to it.[18] But it is thought to have been neglected in an era of nursing shortages and high-tech medicine.

A third perspective relates to the availability and use of complementary therapies in an inpatient setting.[19] The AHA's 2005 survey found that 26.5 percent of hospitals made one or more such therapies available to their patients, an increase from 7.7 percent in 1998.[20] In part, this no doubt reflects a general increase in patient demand for these therapies, even though a recent Institute of Medicine report finds that relatively little research has been conducted to date that assesses their effectiveness.[21]

A fourth perspective concerns the proactive use of various means of spiritual support in the care of receptive patients.[22] This component goes beyond the traditional role of the hospital chaplain and includes training hospital staff to provide spiritual support for patients and family members who request it.

HOW WERE THE STUDY HOSPITALS SELECTED?

In order to address the questions we have posed regarding the efforts of hospitals to reinvent the patient experience, we adopted a multiorganizational case-study research design. (We describe elements of that design, including data collection methods, in the appendix.) We focused on understanding, at a deep level, the efforts of a relatively small number of hospitals. Because we wanted to understand the ways in which hospitals combined different components into a coherent overall strategy for change, we selected hospitals for our study that had implemented broad-based approaches to reinventing the patient experience. The names and selected characteristics of the eight study hospitals are contained in Table 1.1. All but one of these hospitals invested in changes in the physical environment, but there was considerable variation in emphasis placed on the other components (Table 1.2).

In selecting hospitals for inclusion in the study, we also sought variation in characteristics that we expected to influence implementation. In particular, we selected hospitals that varied in size, geographic location, and length of time since they had begun their efforts to change the patient experience. The size of the hospital could influence the strategy adopted, the implementation barriers encountered, and the sustainability of the strategy. For instance, large hospitals may have more resources to devote to organizational change activities, including a greater capacity to support innovation through philanthropy. On the other hand, the influence of a charismatic leader could be felt more readily by everyone in a small hospital but could lose much of its impact if diffused through the administrative bureaucracy of a larger organization.

With respect to region, research has documented that care processes in hospitals vary widely across communities.[23] Also, variation can occur in the functioning of labor markets for hospital employees, community acceptance of nontraditional treatment approaches, the policies of health insurers, and the benefit designs of public and private payers, all of which could shape the environment for the change efforts of hospitals.

The length of time over which hospitals have attempted to implement and sustain their strategies could be an important consideration for several reasons. For instance, an initial spurt of activity could be

Table 1.1. Characteristics of Study Hospitals

Hospital	Affiliation	Number of Beds	Medical Staff (Physicians)	Market	Location	% Revenue from Medicare
Abbott Northwestern Hospital	System	621	1,600	Competitive	Minneapolis, MN	35
Florida Hospital–Celebration Health	System	100	90 *	Competitive	Celebration, FL	36
Highline Medical Center	Independent	176	275	Competitive	Burien, WA	42
North Hawaii Community Hospital	Independent	40	144	Protected	Waimea, HI	30
St. Charles Medical Center–Bend	Independent	216	319	Protected	Bend, OR	42
St. Rose Dominican Hospitals–Siena Campus	System	214	1,000	Competitive	Henderson, NV	29
The Valley Hospital	Independent	451	800	Competitive	Ridgewood, NJ	45
Windber Medical Center	System	82	60	Competitive	Windber, PA	58

* 2,000 across all campuses.

Table 1.2. Components of Consumer-Focused Innovation Strategy

Hospital	Key Event in Strategy Formation	Relative Emphasis on Component			
		Physical Environment	Holistic Nursing	CAM*	Spiritual Support
Abbott Northwestern Hospital	Formation of Institute for Health and Healing (2001) with major donated funding	Medium	Medium	Medium	Low
Florida Hospital–Celebration Health	Construction of new hospital (1997)	High	Low	Low	High
Highline Medical Center	Attendance of administrative staff at conference (1992)	Medium	Medium	Low	Low
North Hawaii Community Hospital	Construction of new hospital (1996) with major donated funding	High	Medium	Medium	Medium
St. Charles Medical Center–Bend	Formalization of Healing Health Care philosophy (early 1990s)	Medium	High	Low	Low
St. Rose Dominican Hospitals–Siena Campus	Construction of new Siena Campus (1998)	High	Low	Low	High
The Valley Hospital	Arrival of new chief nursing officer (1998)	Low	High	Medium	Low
Windber Medical Center	Arrival of new chief executive officer (1997)	Medium	Medium	High	Low

* Complementary and alternative medicine.

supported by a visionary leader. Over time, as leadership changes, the enthusiasm for the change strategy could decline, or the strategy could be reshaped by new leadership. In effect, the experiences of the hospitals, and the challenges they face in sustaining change, could depend on where they are in their own trajectory.

The group of study hospitals does vary along these and other dimensions. Half belong to multihospital systems, two of which have a religious affiliation or sponsorship. Six hospitals are in markets with a large number of diverse competitors, while two are in relatively protected markets. Four hospitals are in the western United States, two in the East, and one each is in the South and Midwest. The hospitals range in size from 40 beds to more than 600 beds and from 60 medical staff members to about 1,600. A similarly wide variation is seen in the study hospitals' dependence on Medicare for inpatient revenues. This variation lets us explore how hospitals of all different types have developed and implemented strategies to reinvent the patient experience.

SUMMARY

We selected eight hospitals for inclusion in this book. They varied along a number of important dimensions that could affect their selection of change strategies and their ability to implement them. Guided by a framework developed from the published literature, we conducted interviews with hospital leadership and analyzed documents pertinent to the hospitals' efforts to reinvent the patient experience (see appendix). In the next eight chapters, we describe the experiences of the eight hospitals in detail.

ENDNOTES

1. Robinson, J. C., and S. Dratler. 2006. "Corporate Structure and Capital Strategy at Catholic Healthcare West." *Health Affairs* 25 (1): 134–47; see esp. 134.

2. Bazzoli, G. J., L. Dynan, L. R. Burns, and C. Hay. 2004. "Two Decades of Organizational Change in Health Care: What Have We Learned?" *Medical Care Research and Review* 61 (3): 247–331.

3. Devers, K., L. Brewster, and L. Casalino. 2003. "Changes in Hospital Competitive Strategy: A New Medical Arms Race?" *Health Services Research* 38 (1): 447–70; Bazzoli, G., A. Gerland, and J. May. 2006. "Construction Activity in U.S. Hospitals." *Health Affairs* 25 (3): 783–91.

4. Appleby, J. 2006. "Hospitals' Profit Margin Hits 6-Year High in 2004." *USA Today* January 5, Money section, 3b.

5. King, J. G., and E. Moran. 2006. "Trust Counts Now. Hospitals and Their Communities." A report to the American Hospital Association. Washington, DC: American Hospital Association; see esp. 3.

6. King and Moran (2006), 3.

7. King and Moran (2006), 5.

8. King and Moran (2006), 5.

9. Robinson, J. C. 2005. "Managed Consumerism in Health Care." Health Affairs 24 (1): 1478–89; Ford, R. C., and M. D. Fottler. 2000. "Creating Customer-Focused Health Care Organizations." *Health Care Management Review* 25 (4): 18–33; Eisenberg, B. 1997. "Customer Service in Healthcare: A New Era." *Hospital and Health Services Administration* 42 (1): 17–31.

10. Shortell, S. M., E. M. Morrison, and B. Friedman. 1990. *Strategic Choices for America's Hospitals: Managing Change in Turbulent Times.* San Francisco: Jossey-Bass, 27–45.

11. Robinson (2005).

12. Lindenauer, P., D. Remus, S. Roman, M. Rothberg, E. Benjamin, A. Ma, and D. Bratzler. 2007. "Public Reporting and Pay for Performance in Hospital Quality Improvement." *New England Journal of Medicine* 356 (5): 486–96; Blank, A. E., S. Horowitz, and D. Matza. 1995. "Quality with a Human Face? The Samuels Planetree Model Hospital Unit." *Journal of Quality Improvement* 21 (6): 289–99; Schweitzer, M., L. Gilpin, and S. Frampton. 2004. "Healing Spaces: Elements of Environmental Design that Make an Impact on Health." *Journal of Alternative and Complementary Medicine* 10 (Suppl. I): S71–S83.

13. Poole, C. D. 1995. "Something Old, Something New: Facility Expansion Emphasizes Holistic Health." *Health Facilities Management* 8 (12): 14–15; Blank, Horowitz, and Matza (1995); Gearon, C. J. 2002. "Planetree (25 Years Older)." *Hospitals and Health Networks* 76 (10): 40–43; Anonymous. 2003. "Designing for Quality: Hospitals Look to the Built Environment to Provide Better Patient Care and Outcomes." *Quality Letter for Healthcare Leaders* 15 (4): 2–13; Stout, G. 1995.

"Patient-Focused Care from the Ground Up." *Journal of Healthcare Resource Management* 13 (2): 17–22; Bilchik, G. S. 2002. "A Better Place to Heal." *Health Forum* 45 (4): 10–15; Geary, H. 2003. "Facilitating an Organizational Culture of Healing in an Urban Medical Center." *Nursing Administration Quarterly* 27 (3): 231–39.

14. Martin, D. P., P. Diehr, D. A. Conrad, J. H. Davis, R. Leickly, and E. B. Perrin. 1998. "Randomized Trial of a Patient-Centered Hospital Unit." *Patient Education and Counseling* 34 (2): 125–33; Boykin, A., S. O. Schoenhofer, N. Smith, J. St. Jean, and D. Aleman. 2003. "Transforming Practice Using a Caring-Based Nursing Model." *Nursing Administration Quarterly* 27 (3): 223–30; Johnson, B. H. 1999. "Family Focus. When Hospitals Put the Emphasis on Patients and Families, Everyone Benefits." *Trustee* 52 (3): 12–15; Swanson, K., and D. Wojnar. 2004. "Optimal Healing Environments in Nursing." *Journal of Alternative and Complementary Medicine* 10 (Suppl. I): S43–S48.

15. Blank, Horowitz, and Matza (1995); Schweitzer, Gilpin, and Frampton (2004).

16. Poole (1995); Blank, Horowitz, and Matza (1995); Gearon (2002); Anonymous (2003); Stout (1995); Bilchik (2002); Geary (2003).

17. Martin et al. (1998); Boykin et al. (2003); Johnson (1999); Swanson and Wojnar (2004).

18. Kitson, A. 2001. "Nursing Leadership: Bringing Caring Back to the Future." *Quality in Health Care* 10 (Suppl. II): ii79–ii84.

19. Sendelbach, S., L. Carikem, J. Lapensky, and V. Kshettry. 2003. "Developing an Integrative Therapies Program in a Tertiary Care Cardiovascular Hospital." *Critical Care Nursing Clinics of North America* 15 (3): 363–72.

20. Ananth, S. 2006. *Health Forum 2005 Complementary and Alternative Medicine Survey of Hospitals: Summary of Results.* Chicago: American Hospital Association (AHA).

21. Ernst, E. 2003. "Complementary Medicine: Where Is the Evidence?" *Journal of Family Practice* 52 (8): 630–34; Institute of Medicine (IOM), Committee on the Use of Complementary and Alternative Medicine. 2005. *Complementary and Alternative Medicine in the United States.* Washington, DC: The National Academies Press; Birch, S., J. K. Besselink, F. A. M. Jonkman, T. A. M. Hekker, and A. Box. 2004. "Clinical Research on Acupuncture: Part 1. What Have Reviews of the Efficacy and Safety of Acupuncture Told Us So Far?" *Journal of Alternative and Complementary Medicine* 10 (3): 468–80.

22. Thornton, L. 2005. "The Model of Whole-Person Caring: Creating and Sustaining a Healing Environment." *Holistic Nursing Practice* 19 (3): 106–15; Luskin, F. 2004. "Transformative Practices for Integrating Mind-Body-Spirit." *Journal of Alternative and Complementary Medicine* 10 (Suppl. I): S15–S23.

23. Wennberg, J. E., E. S. Fisher, T. A. Stukel, and S. M. Sharp. 2004. "Use of Medicare Claims Data to Monitor Provider-Specific Performance among Patients with Severe Chronic Illness." *Health Affairs*. [Online article; retrieved 8/23/06.] content.healthaffairs.org/webexclusives/index.dtl?year=2004.

CHAPTER 2

Windber Medical Center:
Crisis Leads to Change

EXECUTIVE SUMMARY

In 1997, Windber Medical Center (WMC) appeared to have no future as an acute care hospital. Eight years later, it is a thriving, financially viable organization that is a source of great community pride. Many factors have contributed to this dramatic change, but WMC leadership believe that their pursuit of an "integrative healthcare" approach to patient care has been a driving force behind the hospital's recent success. According to WMC, "Integrative healthcare gives people the tools to nurture the connection between the mind and body, empowering people to help heal themselves. Integrative healthcare allows one to develop a partnership with their healthcare team. One can now take an active role in their own business."[1] Pursuing this strategy, WMC has expanded its array of nontraditional services and community outreach activities while at the same time enhancing its use of the newest diagnostic technology. As one leader noted, it has tried to be both high tech and high touch. WMC's integrative care approach has received attention in the national media, for example, in *Forbes* magazine and the *Wall Street Journal,* and WMC's leaders believe this approach is responsible for the very low staff turnover, improved patient care (as evidenced by extremely low

13

infection rates), and increased patient satisfaction. There is a strong belief among WMC's leaders and staff that the direction the hospital has taken over the last few years is not only the right direction to take but also is the likely future for most acute care hospitals operating in an environment that will increasingly demand greater sensitivity and responsiveness to patient preferences. While it has received numerous accolades, WMC continues to face significant day-to-day challenges, not the least of which is how to continue and expand its integrative care approach in the face of limited reimbursements for the nontraditional services it provides.

BACKGROUND

WMC has been in existence for almost 100 years. It is part of the four-hospital Conemaugh Health System, located in west-central Pennsylvania. The flagship hospital in the system, Memorial Medical Center, is a 564-bed (355 in service) facility in Johnstown, Pennsylvania, about 12 miles from WMC. WMC has 82 beds and 450 employees—an increase from 250 employees in 1997—including 60 registered nurses and 25 licensed practical nurses. Approximately 150 physicians are on the medical staff, and about 60 are active participants. The majority of admissions are generated by 30 physicians. WMC owns three primary care practices and employs five obstetricians/gynecologists and a number of emergency department physicians. It also operates an intensive care unit.

At present, approximately 58 percent of WMC's revenue comes from Medicare patients, 25 percent from Highmark Blue Cross Blue Shield (the dominant health plan in the region), and 6 percent from Medicaid. WMC has experienced positive income from operations for each of the last four years, with outpatient revenues increasing by 100 percent in the last five years. Inpatient revenues have been stagnant in a shrinking market. WMC has benefited financially from grant funds from the Department of Defense and donations from other sources.

These funds have been instrumental in supporting the purchase of new technology and the development of new programs.

Several of the financial challenges now facing WMC are similar to those confronting most hospitals of its size. For example, it must set aside increased funds to meet pension obligations and for upkeep and renovation of an aging physical plant. Its medical staff is also growing older on average, and WMC needs to recruit replacement physicians over the coming years. Some of its grant support is ending, so it must now build up reimbursement from private payers for several of its programs. Challenges particular to WMC include a declining population base in its service area (although the low cost of living and availability of veterans' healthcare has attracted some military retirees) and its relationship to the system's flagship hospital. The geographic proximity of WMC to the flagship facility means that, in some respects, this facility is its primary competition for patients. WMC is challenged to maintain a separate identity from the flagship while at the same time being shaped by the overall strategic initiatives of the system.

PURSUING A PATIENT-ORIENTED STRATEGY

The Transition to Integrated Healthcare

When its current president and chief executive officer (CEO) was hired in 1997, WMC was widely believed to be on a rapid downward trajectory that would inevitably end in closure. It had, for a time, been operated as a for-profit facility but then had been turned over to the community without an endowment. Its physical appearance had deteriorated, its medical staff was aging, and it was experiencing difficulty attracting and retaining nursing staff. It did have a new unit with a patient-centered mission to provide palliative care to dying persons, the funds for which had been solicited from the community. It was clear to the new CEO that the hospital would close if dramatic changes were not made.

Making the Hard Decisions

WMC faced significant financial challenges that caused a fundamental rethinking of its mission and business model. F. Nicholas Jacobs, FACHE, describes how he confronted the problems of WMC when he acquired the position of president and CEO:

> The wheels on the bus go round and round, but sometimes the seats are filled with people who thought they were on a horse and buggy.
>
> Upon my arrival at Windber Medical Center, my first two weeks were spent in nearly 300 one-on-one private meetings with our employees. It was a very informative 14-day period of time. In the end, I knew much too much about the facility and its inner workings. In fact, you could ask me just about anything and the answer was on the tip of my newly segmented, mental hard drive.
>
> It was exceedingly clear to me that we had to find a way to deal with each and every issue that had been raised, and it was also abundantly clear that this consideration needed to occur in an expedited manner. Salaries were lagging. Intimate old-boy networks were creating abusive working conditions for those staffers who were not in the club. Most importantly, however, there were at least three dozen people who were not suitable to work in an organization that was attempting to transform itself into one of America's most patient-centered facilities.
>
> Our first center of attention was to the head of the bus, the senior leadership team. Generally, they were a wonderful group of hard-working vice presidents who were firmly ensconced in a world that was very pertinent to 1987, but the problem was that it was 1997. No matter what was suggested at the steering team meetings, they smiled in agreement, left the conference room, and had their private meeting to undermine

the philosophical direction toward which our organization was pointed.

After nearly a year of these passive-aggressive counter-measures, we employed a management consulting behavioral psychologist to analyze the situation and make a presentation to the board that allowed me to begin the transition in senior leadership.

It is with deep embarrassment that I admit that the next crew recruited into these positions, although decades younger, were even less effective. That was probably because they were decades younger, less secure, and more aggressive. The final outcome was the hiring of a group of vice presidents who were predominantly women (mostly new mothers) and a few older men who had impeccable credentials and wonderful nurturing skills. They have been the solution to the problems identified on the first few seats of the bus.

We then launched into an employee evaluation program that helped us identify the 32 highly directive, low-self-image individuals who were incapable of introspection. We then went through a layoff that enabled them to leave with dignity. In fact, we found most of them positions at our competitor's facility.

Since then, we have diligently pursued our goals to hire people who actually like other people. These are people who should be providing care to human beings in need, and the seats are filled with the right people.

The CEO's personal experience caring for his father had convinced him that hospitals tended to serve the needs of the staff more than the needs and preferences of their patients. He saw the approach taken by the palliative care unit, with respect to the way in which patient and family needs were addressed, as a model for the hospital as a whole. With "nothing to lose," as he put it, the new CEO decided to attempt to change the management and culture of the hospital to make it more patient centered and "community oriented." In the first month of his tenure as CEO, WMC affiliated with Planetree, a national organization that emphasizes the patient environment as an important factor in healing. Founded in 1978, Planetree supports pleasant, caring, family-oriented environments for patients and recognizes patient and family rights and responsibilities in the healing process. Planetree hospitals are committed to providing a warm, relaxing, noninstitutional environment for their patients and integrating modern medicine with more traditional practices directed at healing the mind, body, and spirit. (See the Planetree website at www.planetree.org for more information.)

This commitment has resulted in the implementation of a variety of nontraditional patient and community activities by WMC, including yoga, acupuncture, aromatherapy, biofeedback, massage therapy, Reiki, pet therapy, and drumming. A staff person oversees the deployment and management of these programs, their integration with clinical care, and their availability to the community.

The first step in implementing new programs of this type at WMC typically involves securing the support of hospital staff. Staff members are trained in the programs and their potential applications in patient care. In some cases (e.g., aromatherapy, massage therapy), they participate in the activities to experience their benefits. Medical staff are provided with published studies regarding the effectiveness of the therapies and generally become more accepting of the therapies over time as they see benefits for their patients, particularly in the area of pain management.

Occasionally, implementation of new programs as part of WMC's integrative healthcare strategy met with resistance. For example, some community members accused the hospital of supporting Eastern religions when it offered classes in yoga. WMC needed to explain that yoga was not a religion and that it was being used as a stress management technique. WMC also found that a substantial number of staff members were not supportive of the new approach. As a result, it was forced to terminate the contracts of 34 employees over a period of time, including members of the administrative team. They were replaced with employees who were comfortable with the CEO's vision for transforming the hospital. The hospital's board remained supportive of its new CEO during this difficult time, in part because it recognized the need for change if the hospital was to survive.

Developing New Community-Based Programs

A key to WMC's ultimately successful adoption of an integrated healthcare model by was its ability to establish highly visible programs that brought community members into the facility on a regular basis. The two most important programs in this respect have been the Dr. Dean Ornish Program for Reversing Heart Disease and the hospital's HealthStyles facility.

WMC is one of about 23 sites in the United States to offer the Ornish program, which emphasizes moderate exercise, a low-fat nutrition plan, stress management, and group support, with the goal of improving cardiac function and quality of life. WMC initiated the Ornish program in 2000, and 17 groups have completed it. In addition to providing a service to community members, the program attracted grant funds to the hospital to evaluate results.

The second program, HealthStyles, is based in a fitness facility at WMC that contains an indoor walking track, cardiovascular training equipment, strength training equipment, a group exercise space, and a hydrotherapy pool with underwater treadmill. Membership is available to all community residents 14 years of age and older for a very low monthly fee, and hours of operation are tailored to accommodate work schedules. HealthStyles, which currently has 1,200 members, brings people to the hospital, exposes them to some types of integrative care activities (e.g., yoga), and reinforces community support for WMC.

Still Making the Hard Decisions

When WMC began introducing new therapeutic approaches, it met both internal and external resistance. President and CEO F. Nicholas Jacobs, FACHE, discusses how this resistance was overcome:

> Yoga for octogenarians? In 1996 my personal health journey took me to a web page espousing the work of Dr. Dean Ornish and his coronary artery disease reversal program. It was my decision to fly to the Bay area, drop $8,000 from my retirement account, and partake in the newly functioning Ornish program. After meeting numerous people who had been given death sentences a decade and a half earlier but who were still alive and doing well, it was also my decision to bring that program back to our small, urban medical center in south-central Pennsylvania.
>
> Unfortunately, the 800-pound gorilla in Western Pennsylvania health insurance, Highmark Blue Cross, had decided that no hospital was fit to administer this program at that time, and because they had formed a partnership with Dr. Ornish, blocked us from participation in the official Ornish program for several months. (We later came to a settlement and are now one of their demonstration sites nationally as a model for the success of this venture.)
>
> Because we were officially prevented from running an Ornish program, we decided to begin experimenting with segments of the program on our own, segments that were not protected via copyrights, ownership, and the like. Our first dive into the elements of Ornish was to begin yoga classes, but our hospital was 100 years old and did not have appropriate rooms for these types of physical activities. Before long, we struck a deal with two of the four Catholic churches that were within a two-block area of our hospital to allow classes to be held in their recreation and banquet rooms.

Dr. Ornish had repeatedly predicted that his program would fail in a town filled with older, ethnic oriented individuals who had grown up on porkette sandwiches, kolbassi, and meatballs. Imagine my delight when, upon visiting one of the first classes, we saw two dozen men and women in their 60s, 70s, and 80s on the floor doing the gentle bridge yoga position.

About a year after that, our Integrative Health Center was completed, and a group of our most conservative physicians and one chaplain on our staff began to notice that patient-centered care meant giving the patients power that they previously possessed. It was after that discovery that they decided to make a motion at the medical staff meeting to ban spiritual touch in our palliative care unit and to question the use of Eastern religions in our relaxation classes.

Within a week we began seeing letters to the editor regarding the use of Eastern spiritual beliefs in Windber Medical Center's classes, and then we received word that the local Baptist Church was organizing to picket our facility. A local podiatrist also did a television interview regarding the taking of souls in our facility by using Eastern religions in place of traditional Christian religions and, because his name was similar to our nationally recognized heart surgeon, plenty of people were confused.

Bottom line? We stopped using the word "yoga" for a few years and replaced it with relaxation techniques and invited everyone to bring their rosaries or prayer beads if they so desired. We then had the three most vocal critics from our staff experience the program and commissioned them to calm the PR waters. Seven years later, yoga is embraced and a daily part of our integrative health life, along with Reiki, massage, acupuncture, aroma, pet, and music therapy, and we have had approximately 500 individuals go through the program.

Developing New Clinical and Research Programs

At the same time WMC was implementing its new integrative care approach, it was also becoming increasingly high tech. The Joyce Murtha Breast Care Center, which opened in 2001, combines breast care and education on women's health issues under one roof. It has also been used as a site in national clinical trials. In addition, the Windber Research Institute was formed as a biomedical research organization focused on breast cancer, and it has received $60 million in grant funding. Operated in collaboration with Walter Reed Army Medical Center in Washington, DC, the institute has developed a research laboratory and tissue repository for clinical breast cancer research. Work at the institute has enabled WMC to acquire state-of-the-art imaging equipment, including a high-definition magnetic resonance imaging (MRI) system and a positron emission tomography/computed tomography scanner, both of which are available for all patients in the hospital.

CHALLENGES TO THE STRATEGY

While the integrative care model is part of the culture of WMC, maintaining and expanding it is a continual financial challenge. Some of the costs of nontraditional programs have been subsidized by synergies with other hospital activities and by donations and grant funds. Profits generated by an aggressive outreach program for laboratory services have also helped. However, WMC is searching for more stable, ongoing sources of funding. For instance, it has entered into a partnership with Highmark Blue Cross Blue Shield that supports the costs of some participants in the Ornish program. And the fee structures for some integrative health services are being reexamined. During the coming year, all occupational therapy and physical therapy patients will be offered one free treatment by the integrative healthcare department. The expectation is that many will return for additional treatments on a fee basis. The cost structure for the acupuncture program is also being examined, with the hope of spreading the fixed program costs (largely physician salaries) over more patients.

Because of the declining population base in the area and the location nearby of a large tertiary hospital in the same healthcare system, opportunity is limited to subsidize integrated healthcare programs with profits generated through inpatient care. The presence of WMC within the larger hospital system also poses other challenges. In a sense, WMC functions as the system's "laboratory" for nontraditional programs. Some programs developed at WMC have been implemented in other system hospitals in some form. Thus, WMC is continually challenged to maintain the unique identity it has established in its market area. According to one WMC leader, the effort to maintain its identity requires that WMC staff remain passionate about providing the best possible patient experience: "When patients come they feel they are important and cared for." The support of the next generation of WMC leaders for the integrative care model will likely determine if it becomes firmly embedded in the hospital's culture.

KEYS TO SUCCESS

WMC's success to date in implementing a patient-centered, integrated care approach in a resource-constrained environment is the result of several key factors, in the opinion of WMC leaders.

Presence of a Significant External Threat

The hospital faced an extreme external threat in 1997 that was acknowledged by most people employed in the facility, the hospital's board, and the community. The need for change of some type was obvious. This provided the new CEO with considerable leverage in implementing his vision for WMC.

Willingness to Make Difficult Decisions

Fairly early in the transition process it became evident that some hospital employees and medical staff were not comfortable with the new patient-centered approach and its emphasis on mind/body/spirit healing. Rather than helping the transition, they became obstacles to it. They were replaced by individuals who were committed to the new vision for WMC. From that point, an important part of the hiring process involved determining the enthusiasm of potential employees for the integrated healthcare approach. As a result, hospital employees, including nurses and, for the most part, medical staff, are now committed to integrated healthcare and to improving patient experiences at WMC.

Ability to Build Community Support

Initially, some in the community were suspicious of the new programs being implemented in the hospital. Personal experience with the programs, word-of-mouth transmission of information in the community, and the enthusiasm of hospital staff were all important in allaying people's concerns. Also, as the hospital's financial situation stabilized and employment at WMC grew, the importance of WMC to the local economy became increasingly evident. Finally, WMC leaders consciously designed programs that would draw community members to the facility and expose them to nontraditional programs. The result was that WMC was transformed in the eyes of community members from a community "failure" to a valued asset deserving of financial and political support.

Balanced Approach to Transformation

WMC's leaders recognized early in the transformation process that, while adopting an integrated healthcare approach was the right thing to do for patients and staff, it should proceed in tandem with efforts to enhance medical treatment. The ability to do this, through grants and the establishment of the breast center and the research institute, created a more accepting environment for implementing of nontraditional programs.

ENDNOTE

1. Windber Medical Center (WMC), Institute of Integrative Medicine. 2007. "Healing Body, Mind & Spirit." [Online information; retrieved 3/7/07.] www.windbercare.com/inthealth.asp.

CHAPTER 3

St. Rose Dominican Hospitals–Siena Campus: Creating a New Environment for Hospital Care

EXECUTIVE SUMMARY

St. Rose Dominican Hospitals–Siena Campus (SRDHSC) opened its doors in 2000 to serve the rapidly growing population around Henderson, Nevada. SRDHSC also provided an opportunity for the Adrian Dominican Sisters to continue and extend their service mission to the community while at the same time creating a physical environment supportive of the organization's belief in a comprehensive mind/body/spirit approach to healing. According to the president of St. Rose Dominican Hospitals (SRDH) and SRDHSC, "Medical science is now confirming what the Adrian Dominican Sisters have always promoted. When helping patients to achieve good health or recover from illness or injury, you must do more than address physical concerns. The health of the mind and spirit are key to overall well being."[1] The opening of this new facility, with design features intended to support a healing environment for patients, coincided with major initiatives from Catholic Healthcare West (CHW), of which SRDH is an affiliate, that focused on improving the patient experience. SRDHSC's leaders believe that the mission, vision, and values that the Dominican Sisters have long espoused for SRDH, combined with the healing environment in SRDHSC, have created an important model for hospitals nationally, as well as a unique niche for SRDH in the communities it serves. However, they face challenges with this model. The number of sisters is declining, which raises concerns about sustaining their vision and values into the future. And population growth is straining the capacity of SRDHSC and its staff, at times making it difficult to maintain the quality of the patient experience.

BACKGROUND

The Rose de Lima Campus, SRDH's original facility, was built in 1942 by the U.S. government and acquired by the Dominican Sisters of Adrian, Michigan, in 1947. Responding to growth of the surrounding community, the hospital grew in size and technological sophistication over the years. In 1988, it joined CHW. Formed in 1986 and headquartered in San Francisco, CHW is currently a system of 40 hospitals and medical centers in Arizona, Nevada, and California. It is the eighth largest hospital system in the United States and now includes both religious and secular hospitals. Even with the addition of secular facilities, CHW continues to affirm its commitment to "compassionate, high quality, affordable health care services in a compassionate environment that is attuned to every patient's physical, mental and spiritual needs."[2] At the Rose de Lima Campus, a major four-story expansion was completed in 1991, and in 1998 ground was broken for SRDH's Siena Campus, which added 214 beds to the 138 beds of the original Rose de Lima Campus.

SRDHSC offers a broad range of high-tech hospital services, including a pediatric intensive care unit (ICU), an open-heart surgery center, neurosurgery, a Level II nursery, obstetrical services, and state-of-the-art digital diagnostic imaging. SRDH now has more than 2,000 employees, including 700 to 800 nurses, across both campuses and approximately 1,000 physicians on the medical staff. Between 200 and 250 of these physicians do 90 percent or more of their work at the SRDH campuses. Nurses move between the two campuses as needed. At present, 21.3 percent of SRDH's revenues come from Medicare, 4.4 percent from Medicaid, and 74.3 percent from all other payer sources, including insurance and self-pay. SRDH reportedly contributes more than $32 million annually to charity care and to community programs.

SRDH competes for patients in the greater Las Vegas area. This market is served by three systems: HCA (which has three hospitals in the area), Universal Health (four hospitals), and Iasis (one hospital). University Medical Center also has a significant presence in the market, but SRDH does not regard it as a direct competitor. These organizations compete for patients during the warm months, but the increased population in the area during the cooler months means that all hospitals operate at or near capacity. SRDHSC averages a 90 percent occupancy rate but is 100 percent occupied during some periods in the winter, stressing the capacity of the facility and its emergency department. SRDH is the only religious, not-for-profit hospital organization in the southern part of Nevada and differentiates itself from its competitors in this respect. In outward appearance, the physical plant on each campus underscores this difference, with a cross on top of each facility and a religious statue at the main entrance.

Soon after SRDHSC opened, it was operating at close to full capacity. In response, in February 2004 SRDH broke ground for a third acute care facility—the San Martín Campus—located in southwest Las Vegas. San Martín offers 111 private rooms and has the ability to expand by 90 private rooms in the future. A three-story medical office building was also constructed as part of the project. The San Martín Campus, like SRDHSC, is designed to create a physical environment for patients that supports a mind/body/spirit approach to healing.

SRDH has developed a large number of innovative programs that address community needs outside the walls of its inpatient facilities. The nature of these programs is a direct reflection of SRDH's mission statement, "Under the sponsorship of the Adrian

Dominican Sisters and in response to the changing needs of the people of southern Nevada, St. Rose Dominican Hospitals offer quality, compassionate care. We promote wholeness of body, mind and spirit in the Dominican tradition of working with others to improve the health status of the community in a shared pursuit for justice and truth with a commitment to those with special needs."[3]

Programs run the gamut from education to support groups to direct care. For example, in 1998 it established, through an endowment gift, the Barbara Greenspun WomensCare Center of Excellence. The center has an educational mission, offering classes in exercise, nutrition, and parenting; maintains a lending library; and publishes *WomensCare* magazine, which reaches about 360,000 households.

SRDH facilitates support groups in areas such as alcoholism, bereavement, breast cancer, depression, diabetes, divorce, eating disorders, fibromyalgia, gambling addiction, narcotics, infertility, and pregnancy loss. It operates a variety of community outreach programs, many focused on the healthcare needs of the disadvantaged. One example is its Positive Impact Program, which provides medical and dental services to children in more than 60 local schools who are referred by school nurses. Students meeting eligibility criteria are provided with healthcare at no cost. The program is funded through donations of medical services and money. All of its outreach programs are seen as consistent with the mission of serving the healthcare needs of the community, in addition to the needs of patients admitted to SRDH.

PURSUING A PATIENT-ORIENTED STRATEGY

The leadership of SRDH has pursued a multifaceted approach in an attempt to create and support an environment conducive to mind/body/spirit healing for patients. Each of the different facets is described in the following sections, focusing on SRDHSC.

Physical Environment

SRDHSC was designed to be a soothing, patient- and family-friendly environment. For example, it contains a three-quarter-acre healing garden with flowing water, sunlight, plants, and a rose-covered gazebo. All rooms are private and include family space to encourage family participation in the healing process. Carpeting in the hallways helps muffle sound, and soothing music is part of the overall environment. Each floor has quiet rooms for patients and visitors, and no overhead paging is done except in emergencies. Arches with inspirational quotations painted above them are used to connect parts of the facility, and the overall design makes use of natural light wherever possible.

Starting from the Ground Up

"Gathering input from staff and physicians about building a new healthcare facility is as important as consulting your family when designing a new home. Feeling comfortable in your space is critical," says Vicky VanMeetren, CEO of SRDH–San Martín Campus. She has provided leadership for building more than one hospital from the ground up. She starts with a survey process to ask staff and physicians, "What does *healing environment* mean to you?"

"It's interesting," she says. "People start by answering that question from the perspective of their work role—nurse, physician, housekeeper. But inevitably, they end up giving feedback from a more personal viewpoint. Everyone has been a patient at some time in his or her life." VanMeetren's most recent building, SRDHSC in Henderson, Nevada, is a model facility for healing, and much attention was paid to staff-inspired details. "Certain spaces absolutely scream of healing to us. One of the most important spaces is the actual patient room. It has become very clear to me that the patient's room is really divided into three types of space: space for the patient, space for the clinician, and very clearly a space for the family. I think that in this day and age, if you try to take that family space and minimize it in any way, then you're not going to meet the patients' needs. The hospital stay is getting shorter, and to welcome a family member into the care if they want to be involved is essential to the patients' actual recovery after they get home."

In designing these healing environments, VanMeetren and her team have incorporated ecumenical chapels, private hallways that provide patient dignity during transport, carpeted ICUs with propel-assisted gurneys, donor-initiated healing gardens, art, and an aquarium filled with handblown glass sculptures and exotic fish in the emergency department waiting room, a nice contrast to most waiting room spaces, which typically display loud televisions.

According to VanMeetren, "you absolutely must have a blend of [architectural] expertise on the build side, as well as the expertise of the people who will use the space. It's often one person's idea that makes a tremendous difference."

Spiritual Emphasis

SRDHSC has a chapel in which Mass takes place on a regularly scheduled basis. A cross and a copy of SRDH's mission statement are prominently placed on the wall of each patient room. Nurses are encouraged to stop and talk or pray with patients and families. It is CHW's policy that each hospital has a spiritual care leader who is responsible for developing and maintaining a comprehensive program of spiritual care. The spiritual care team is charged with helping patients "integrate their spiritual values and beliefs to promote healing…and alleviate suffering."[4] At SRDHSC, spiritual interventions are documented in the patient's medical record, and a member of the spiritual care team responds to each emergency in the facility.

The Spiritual Dimension of Healing

When asked to share some key aspects of her organization's corporate strategy for delivering spiritual care in CHW hospitals at a time when budgets are tight and expectations for productivity are high, Rey Friel, vice president of Mission Integration and Spiritual Care for CHW, responded:

> The strategy comes out of a core belief that healing, of its nature, includes a spiritual dimension. If we really want to be healers in the world and in our communities, then we have to include spiritual care as the hallmark of our care.
>
> We have found that people can find spirituality in so many ways. We often describe spirituality as "that which gives you meaning and purpose in life." Spirituality can also be described as the characteristics and qualities of one's relationship with the Transcendent. Rabbi Abraham Heschel, a well-known writer, philosopher, and teacher, says that "in order to heal a person, we must first be a person." Robots running machines don't heal people. We need to be connected with our own sense of meaning, purpose, transcendence, and community—and not shut off when we act as healers for others.
>
> One of the ways CHW sustains a values-based culture, especially within a secular business model, is through a program called the Ministry Leadership Center. Participants in this three-year program engage in a formative learning experience with their peers around topics such as vocation, heritage, suffering, and social justice. Sessions include two-day, off-site retreats held four times a year, monthly meetings with "dialog partners," and assignments designed to facilitate the integration of learning into leadership in the workplace. Upon completing the three-year program, graduates will become mentors for the next group of leaders.
>
> During the program, participants explore questions such as, "What is the difference between *job, career,* and *calling*?"

"How do we apply Catholic social teaching in a pluralistic society?" "How do we draw on the wisdom of our heritage to find answers to issue we are facing today?" "How do we nurture a values-based culture?" and "How do we sustain that culture over time—when leadership and other events change the cultural landscape almost daily?"

It's that kind of formation experience that we are focused on. Like walking a labyrinth, you go into the center, but then you need to come out again. Participants go away for retreat and reflection, and then go back to the workplace to act from a new perspective. I've heard some of my colleagues remark, "Hey—I'm 50 years old! Why didn't I ever pay attention to this stuff before?" Our teacher gently reminds us that "in spiritual learning, time doesn't matter. Learning the ways of the Spirit can take a lifetime, or it can happen in a single moment."

Patient Satisfaction Initiatives

Under its current patient satisfaction initiative, CHW challenges affiliated hospitals to compete for rewards of $250,000 each, which can be used for whatever purposes are deemed appropriate by the winning hospitals. Hospitals are judged according to patient responses in satisfaction surveys, in which they are asked whether they are likely to return to the hospital and whether they will recommend the hospital to a friend. Hospital employees are also part of a "patient recovery" initiative, whereby they are authorized to take immediate action to help patients recover from any bad service experience they may have had in the hospital. All new employees are educated in the patient satisfaction program, and reeducation occurs periodically. At SRDHSC, it was reported that some nurses were not comfortable with the heavy emphasis on patient satisfaction and moved to other facilities. Nevertheless, in general, the patient satisfaction program is regarded positively by employees, and leaders believe it has helped make SRDH the first choice for nurses seeking employment in the area and has been an important factor in nurse retention. SRDH attempts to hire nurses who have the personality and the values that make them comfortable working in an environment that emphasizes a mind/body/spirit approach to healing. As a result, nurses at SRDH now regard treating the mind, body, and spirit as simply the right thing to do, and the leadership reports a high level of satisfaction among the nursing staff.

CHALLENGES TO THE STRATEGY

At present, SRDH appears to be operating in a community and a corporate environment that are very supportive of its emphasis on mind, body, and spirit in treating hospitalized patients, and its commitment to community outreach programs. However, hospital leaders express three concerns—two immediate and one looming. An immediate concern is the rapid population growth in Las Vegas. While this benefits SRDH (as described later), it has also created periods during which the hospital operates at capacity. This increases the demands on staff and the level of stress they experience. Less time is available to spend in conversation with patients and families, and staff may become less attentive to patient needs. Leaders hope that the opening of the San Martín Campus will alleviate some of the demand at SRDHSC; however, this is likely to be a short-term effect, if it occurs at all. San Martín is not located near Siena, and the continued population growth in Las Vegas is likely to quickly fill any empty Siena beds.

A second immediate concern is the ability of SRDH to attract sufficient numbers of nursing and technical employees who share its mission, vision, and values. This is especially important given the increased need for trained staff generated by the opening of the San Martín Campus. While Las Vegas is attracting large numbers of retirees, its image is not always attractive to young professionals with families who want to put down roots in a community.

Finally, a longer-term concern expressed by SRDH leaders relates to the decline in the numbers of Adrian Dominican Sisters. Currently, the sisters are very active and visible on the two campuses. Their presence reinforces the emphasis on the spiritual aspects of healing, and SRDH will be challenged to sustain this emphasis as the number of sisters involved in the hospitals decreases.

KEYS TO SUCCESS

SRDH's success to date in developing an integrated mind/body/spirit approach to healing, as exemplified on its Siena Campus, is attributed by its leaders to a variety of factors, some external to SRDH, and others internal.

Rapid Population Growth in the Community

Paradoxically, while rapid population growth has challenged SRDH in some respects, it has supported a mind/body/spirit approach in others. Most importantly, it has ensured a steady demand for the high-tech care available at SRDH. The revenues generated through the provision of this care have kept the hospital in a strong financial position. This has enabled the hospital to invest in community outreach initiatives, implement internal programs supporting patients and families, and construct new campuses designed to support mind/body/spirit healing.

Construction of New Physical Plant

The ability to construct new campuses designed specifically to support a mind/body/spirit approach to healing has allowed SRDH to fully implement its mission and values at the patient bedside. It has enhanced the experience of both staff and patients and, in the opinion of leadership, has resulted in greater staff satisfaction, which in turn has led to better patient care.

Congruence of Values

The mission and values of CHW and of SRDH are largely congruent. This is illustrated clearly in the patient satisfaction program developed at the corporate level. The objectives of this program are consistent with the goals of SRDH with respect to its patients. Support has been provided at the corporate level for the program, and an SRDH employee has been given the responsibility for managing the patient satisfaction initiative at the corporate level.

Unique Market Position

The fact that SRDH is the only not-for-profit, religious-sponsored hospital in the area creates an advantage in two ways. Most obviously, it is the only option for patients who value these characteristics in their choice of hospital. Also, importantly, it is the only alternative for medical and nursing staff who seek these characteristics in their work environment. People with this orientation select into employment at SRDH in part because there are no similar local alternatives. Overall, the unique market position of SRDH has contributed to the creation of a loyal patient and employee base that is fully supportive of its mission, vision, and values.

ENDNOTES

1. Saint Rose Dominican Hospitals (SRDH). 2007. "Serving the Henderson and Las Vegas Communities." [Online information; retrieved 4/18/07.] www.strosehospitals.org.

2. Catholic Healthcare West (CHW). 2007. "CHW at a Glance." [Online information; retrieved 4/18/07.] www.chwhealth.org

3. SRDH. 2007. "Mission statement." [Online information; retrieved 3/7/07.] www.strosehospitals.org/stellent/websites/get_page_cache.esp?nodeId=5001331.

4. CHW. 2007. "Benchmarks for Spiritual Care." [Online information; retrieved 4/18/07.] www.chwhealth.org.

CHAPTER 4

Abbott Northwestern Hospital: Combining High Tech and High Touch

EXECUTIVE SUMMARY

Abbott Northwestern Hospital (ANW), located in central Minneapolis, is the flagship hospital of Allina Hospitals and Clinics, a not-for-profit healthcare system with primary operations in the Minneapolis–St. Paul area. A large, technologically sophisticated enterprise, ANW has fostered initiatives in its inpatient and outpatient care units that promote and support a mind/body/spirit approach to healthcare. These initiatives have been supported by a newly constructed heart hospital, the Institute for Health and Healing (formed in 2002), and the Virginia Piper Cancer Institute.

The primary challenges facing ANW have been how to reconcile mind/body/spirit approaches to healing with ANW's traditionally high-tech culture, how to integrate these approaches into everyday hospital operations, and how to fund them on an ongoing basis. ANW has responded by implementing a "consultative model," with the institute as the centerpiece. Institute consultations may be ordered by any member of the patient's healthcare team, including the patient or a family member. (Acupuncture consultations can be ordered only by a physician.) These services include, but are not limited to, massage therapy, aromatherapy, biofeedback-guided imagery, and music therapy.

An institute practitioner assesses the patient's condition, explains the services available, and work with the patient and the healthcare team to develop a plan for incorporating specific services into the patient's overall treatment.

Acceptance of this approach by the medical and nursing staff has been growing, as has the number of patients receiving services through the institute. However, successfully managing the process of integrating a high-touch patient care approach into the high-tech environment of a major tertiary hospital has been, and continues to be, challenging. It has required the ongoing support of upper-level management, continuous education of medical and nursing staff, and significant subsidies from hospital benefactors.

BACKGROUND

Allina Hospitals and Clinics consists of nine hospitals in Minnesota and western Wisconsin, the Phillips Eye Institute, and 30 clinics. ANW is the largest hospital in the system, with 621 beds, 5,200 employees, more than 1,600 physicians on its medical staff, and operating revenues of $655 million in 2004. Approximately 2,000 nurses are employed by ANW, 60 percent of whom work part time (defined as fewer than 32 hours per week). Union contracts covering hospital nurses provide full-time benefits for employment at 16 hours or more per week. The nurse vacancy rate is about 4 percent.

ANW is organized according to ten centers of excellence, ranging from the world-famous Sister Kenney Rehabilitation Institute to the nationally renowned cardiovascular heart center. ANW was ranked the 25th best hospital for heart care and heart surgery by *U.S. News and World Report* in 2005 and was ranked in the top 50 in four other areas. It has 19 separate departments/programs and provides a full range of outpatient services in addition to its new heart hospital.

Because it is located just south of downtown Minneapolis, ANW competes directly with several other sophisticated tertiary hospitals, including Fairview/University of Minnesota, Fairview Southdale, Methodist Hospital, and North Memorial. All of these hospitals are in greater Minneapolis; ANW does not view itself as competing with non-Allina hospitals in St. Paul. A relatively new hospital in suburban St. Paul, owned by a St. Paul–based hospital system, also provides programs to patients that promote a mind/body/spirit approach to healing, carried out in a supportive physical environment. Because of its location, its considerably smaller size, and the more limited range of services it offers, ANW does not regard this hospital as a direct competitor.

The medical and nursing staffs of ANW have undergone considerable stress as the result of implementing an electronic medical record (EMR) system in the facility. Net operating revenue declined in 2005, caused in part by declines in productivity due to staff time devoted to EMR implementation efforts. Problems with the system have caused some medical staff defections and created challenges to traditional physician/nurse communication. Also, as expected, implementing the EMR system has consumed substantial financial resources in the hospital, as well as the time of hospital managers.

Implementing the EMR system is complicated by the fact that the hospital is in the process of recruiting a new CEO. When the new CEO is hired, he or she will be the third person to fill that position in the last six years. Changeover at the CEO position has created the need for continued efforts (successful to this point) to maintain the support of hospital administration for mind/body/spirit healing initiatives. The president and CEO of Allina has been instrumental in providing continuing support for the institute's work.

PURSUING A PATIENT-ORIENTED STRATEGY

Impetus for Adopting a Mind/Body/Spirit Approach to Healing

When the Virginia Piper Cancer Institute was established at ANW, it incorporated a healing arts program that included massage therapy, acupuncture, a healing coach, and group support for cancer patients. These therapies were made available to help patients cope with the pain and depression that often accompany a diagnosis of cancer. Currently, the cancer institute provides a "healing coach" to patients at their request. The coach helps the patient develop a healing plan and "bridge the worlds of mainstream and complementary medicine."[1] Therapies available to cancer patients include acupuncture, massage, therapeutic touch, and "mind-body skills," all offered through the hospital's Institute for Health and Healing.

The focus of the hospital's efforts to create an optimal healing environment for patients was extended in 2002 to include the formation of the Institute for Health and Healing within the hospital. The inspiration for this new direction was provided by North Hawaii Community Hospital, which had been established under the leadership of Earl Bakken, the founder of Medtronic, a major medical device company located in the Twin Cities. The chairman of the board of Allina at that time succeeded Bakken as the CEO of Medtronic. At this person's urging, the hospital sent a delegation to North Hawaii Community Hospital with a goal of better understanding its philosophy and operations. The CEO of ANW became an advocate and a spokesperson for the formation of the institute, and the family foundation of Allina's board chairman contributed $2 million for start-up costs. (North Hawaii Community Hospital is profiled in Chapter 8.)

Using Philanthropy to Support Change

Philanthropists have played a key role in ANW's ability to pursue high-touch, along with high-tech, treatment approaches. Sid Mallory, president of Abbott Northwestern Hospital Foundation, describes how this was accomplished:

> Since its founding in 2003, the success of the Institute for Health and Healing has been exceptional. In the inpatient setting, the institute's practitioners provide an average of 1,000

patient visits per month, averaging three visits per patient. The outpatient center has exceeded budgeted projections every month since opening in July 2004. The institute was founded with two major lead gifts from Penny and Bill George and the George Family Foundation and Roberta Mann-Benson and the Ted and Roberta Mann Foundation.

The vision for the Institute for Health and Healing is to be a national model of whole-person, patient-centered care. It operates in three areas:

Clinical Services: The institute has an outpatient clinic as well as services for inpatients, including holistic nursing, a healing coach, an outpatient physician, and complementary/alternative medicine practitioners, including acupuncture, nutrition, massage, reflexology, and healing touch.

Education: Education of clinicians is key to the vision of integrative medicine—to incorporate the practice and philosophy into the standard of care at Abbott Northwestern, and to truly "plant" the program into the way we provide clinical care every day and in every center of excellence.

Research: The institute is conducting research into the effectiveness of integrative care in patient outcomes and building a business case for support both within the hospital and with third-party payers.

This project is a great example of bringing the community together to meet a need that only philanthropy could achieve. There is limited reimbursement available today for inpatient integrative therapies. The vision of the institute can only be achieved with philanthropic funding from our community.

The Abbott Northwestern Hospital Foundation has set a goal of raising $15 million and has recruited a steering committee of community volunteers to help educate the community and raise the needed seed philanthropic funding. As of November 1, 2006, more than $7.5 million has been raised. The committee continues to identify and solicit new prospects in the community.

This donation was matched by a contribution from a second foundation, providing the basis for ongoing fund-raising. As part of the design process for the institute, information was gathered from hospitals across the country regarding comparable initiatives. This exploratory process suggested that, at that time, most innovative hospitals in the area of mind/body/spirit approaches to healing were small. ANW felt that it would need to invent a model for the institute that would work in a large, complex tertiary facility.

As the mission and structure for the institute evolved, hospital administration saw it as an organizational response to patient desires for care that was more "relationship centered." In addition to providing better care and a better experience for patients, the hospital hoped that the institute and its efforts would differentiate ANW from its competitors and help attract and retain patients and staff. The leadership harbored no expectation at this early stage that it would reduce hospital costs immediately, and it maintained a belief that the hospital would need to subsidize the institute's efforts through fund-raising. However, a process was established to collect data that could be used to assess the impact of an integrative approach to care on length of stay in the hospital and patient and staff satisfaction.

An important early activity in developing the institute involved holding focus groups within each of the hospital's centers of excellence. These focus groups uncovered many different and uncoordinated efforts to provide alternative care to patients. While the need for better coordination was clear, the focus groups also suggested that staff were cautious of implementing a new initiative. They were concerned about how it would affect their patients and somewhat apprehensive that it would impose new, work-related demands. The focus-group findings suggested that the hospital would need to engage in a carefully planned effort to bring medical and nursing staff on board if the institute was to be a success. Hospital leaders convened a mandatory Saturday retreat for physician leaders at a local spa (the institute was not yet functioning). At this retreat, physicians experienced a variety of alternative and complementary care modalities and discussed how they could be used in treating patients. Once the institute was established, a similar half-day session was conducted in the hospital for nursing leaders, with the same objective. In retrospect, the institute believes that these programs were, and continue to be, essential in building internal support and addressing the concerns of skeptics.

Care Delivery at the Institute for Health and Healing

According to ANW, the Institute for Health and Healing "provides integrative medicine at Abbott Northwestern Hospital, both for inpatients and at an outpatient center. Integrative medicine blends the best of conventional medicine with healing philosophies and a variety of healing therapies. These therapies, often drawn from other medical traditions, emphasize caring for the whole person and focus on healing as much as curing....The Institute for Health and Healing recognizes the value of conventional medicine in treating many chronic and acute conditions, as well as its limits when dealing with the complex needs of patients."[2] The mission of the institute is, in part, to "develop innovative, proactive models of care that embrace the strengths of the whole person—body, mind, and spirit—and the families and communities in which we live; and that promote an understanding of the interdependent nature of healing by strengthening the bonds of caregivers with patients and their families."[3]

The institute hired its first nurse clinician in the first quarter of 2003. Its practice model was to have a team serving each center of excellence that consisted of (1) a nurse clinician with a background in providing care to the types of patients treated in that center (e.g., cancer) and training in complementary/alternative medicine (CAM) practices, (2) a massage therapist with experience treating people with medical problems, and (3) an acupuncturist. The team was structured in this way for several reasons. With respect to including a nurse, it was felt that, if care was to be integrated at the bedside, nurse involvement was essential. A massage therapist was included on the team because this type of therapy was well accepted by clinicians as an effective means to relieve pain and stress. Similarly, acupuncture was accepted as an effective pain treatment by most clinicians, and an acupuncturist was already practicing on the hospital's campus.

Currently, the institute manages six teams consisting of 18 full-time practitioners and additional part-time employees. A music therapist is also on staff. The nurses on the team spend about 50 percent of their time in direct patient care and the rest in developing curricula and educating other nurses, healthcare providers, and community members. All nurses in the hospital receive 40 hours of training with five modules, including holistic nursing, massage techniques, guided imagery, relaxation techniques, and an overview of aromatherapy and acupuncture. It is anticipated and accepted that some nurses may not be comfortable with this approach and may leave the hospital.

The number of requests for consultations received by the institute has grown steadily over the last two years, despite the disruption that was caused by implementing the EMR system. In 2003, when the teams were first formed, only five physicians at ANW were referring patients to the institute for consultation. Now, 400 physicians (of approximately 1,600 on staff) utilize the institute. On average, the first team provided about 150 patient visits per month. Now, about 1,200 are provided. Massage therapy or acupuncture is provided in approximately 60 percent of these visits. Referrals can come to the institute in a variety of ways, in addition to those made directly by clinicians treating patients. For instance, on the hospital's patient intake form, a question is asked about alternative therapies and if the patient has any experience with them. At this time, the referral can come from the intake nurse at the request of the patient or at the urging of the family. Or if a clinician contacts the institute about an incoming patient who has an interest in alternative therapies, an assessment can be scheduled prior to admittance, to be carried out after admittance. The age of the physician does not seem related to the likelihood of referrals, but specialty does; internists, oncologists, cardiologists, and hospitalists are the most likely to refer. Cardiologists frequently offer their patients stress-management therapies and massage. In general, across all therapies, more women than men receive treatments through the institute, and women often request treatment for their spouses.

CHALLENGES TO THE STRATEGY

The efforts of institute staff and others to secure acceptance within ANW of an integrative approach to care and support for the development of a healing environment have been rewarded with significant gains in a relatively short time.

Managing Up

Developing and maintaining a significant high-touch presence in a major medical center can be daunting. Lori Knutson, director of ANW's Institute for Health and Healing, describes her management approach in meeting this challenge:

> Managing up requires an understanding by the one managing up, that integrity and the development of mutually respectful relationships is what allows for an openness for

change, and for ongoing support when times get tough. Leaders are as dependent on dynamic and creative employees as are employees dependent on leaders who take action and have an openness to listen to those who are closest to the work. This mutual and mature understanding is developed through knowledge of human dynamics, intuition, and action. Often what stunts the ability to manage up is fear and lack of self-trust. In other words, managing up requires that one has a confidence in her assessment, evaluation, and plan in order to move forward.

Expressing oneself with conviction and articulating in the language of the organization is essential to being heard. It is also important to acknowledge, outwardly, when actions faltered. Again, honesty creates a firm foundation in the "managing up" relationship. In the realm of integrative medicine, as a paradigm shift in healthcare, there is a foundational skill one must use and enhance in order to accomplish successful managed-up relationships. This skill is a heightened sense for opportunity. Fully understanding senior management, organizational vision, and gaps in the attainment of the vision provides one with the platform by which to build the structure for transformation. The person who is managing up must also have a passion for the vision and a willingness to invest personal time and energy in key organizational relationships and develop the hardiness of detachment to the perceived outcome.

Managing up requires involvement in projects and committees that may not have a direct relationship with moving integrative medicine forward, at least as one sees it at the moment. Involvement in organizational activities provides visibility in the system and gives senior leaders an opportunity to see one [person] beyond the focused position or role. This creates an avenue for exposure and reflects a commitment to the organization as a whole, and not just in relationship to one's personal agenda. This also feeds awareness of what the organization is challenged with and where opportunity lends itself. In managing up it is vital to see the organization from a broad perspective to grasp as many aspects (relationships, resources, wants, and needs) of the organization as possible. Continual objective assessment and evaluation of these aspects will lead to more opportunities to understand when and how to manage up, to build upon change, and to sustain current endeavors.

Finally, managing up requires a clear commitment to oneself, both personally and professionally. Self-care and introspection are essential as one will be challenged physically, emotionally, and spiritually in the process of managing up. Personal health is the cornerstone to successful managing-up relationships. Modeling what one expects to see within the organization will reflect to senior leaders that sense of integrity, which may be the most imperative component in managing up.

However, building on this initial success clearly will be challenging, for several reasons. Certainly, not the least of these is the size and complexity of the hospital. It is difficult to diffuse the current approach throughout the hospital with the available resources. In addition, a number of ongoing issues, while not unusual in a complex hospital, make diffusion more difficult. For example, relations between the hospital and its nurses' union have been difficult in the past year. And, as already noted, the entire hospital has been immersed in implementing an EMR system. Furthermore, turnover at the CEO level within ANW has affected efforts at diffusion. All of these issues together create an environment in which maintaining momentum for the integrative healing approach has required leadership within the institute that understands the challenges of operating in the ANW setting.

A second critical challenge has been financial. Inpatients do not pay out-of-pocket fees for the institute services they receive.

The hospital subsidizes approximately $1 million per year in salaries and secures funding through an additional $700,000 in donations. With respect to outpatient care, revenue is about 50 percent greater than anticipated due in part to the willingness of large health plans in the Twin Cities to reimburse for some of the institute's services, such as acupuncture, nutrition therapy, health coaching, and biofeedback therapy. Outpatient services are expected to reach a break-even point within the next year. However, on the inpatient side, some subsidy through philanthropy will likely always be needed. The institute is now working with the hospital's finance office to develop a business case for the services it provides to hospitalized patients. The hope is that hospital expenses within specific diagnosis-related groups will be reduced because, due to the institute's services, length of stay will be shortened and the use of some classes of drugs, such as narcotics, will be reduced.

KEYS TO SUCCESS

While ANW is still in the very early stage of implementing an integrated mind/body/spirit approach to healthcare within its facility, it has experienced some success in its approach to date, despite the complexity of the implementation environment. This success can be attributed to several factors.

Sponsorship by Key Decision Makers

The strong support of Allina's board chairman, and subsequently of ANW's CEO at the time, was critical to ANW's decision to pursue an integrative approach. There is general agreement that without the interest and support of the chairman, ANW would not have adopted this strategy.

Financial Support Through Philanthropy

The board chairman's family foundation, along with the foundation of another prominent donor, provided substantial start-up funding for the venture. Not only did this allow the hiring of needed staff but it also signaled, in a highly visible way, that the initiative was supported at the highest levels of the organization. The ANW Foundation committee also works to raise funds specifically for the Institute for Health and Healing.

Use of a Consultative Model

The institute employs a model for integrating alternative care into the treatment process that is familiar to clinicians and a good fit with the culture of a large tertiary hospital. It is based on a formal referral process in which clinicians refer patients for consultations with institute staff.

Phased Implementation

In the opinion of institute managers, a very important factor in their success to date has been their ability to convince clinicians that patients can benefit from alternative types of care. An essential aspect of this approach has been the institute's educational workshops and retreats for clinicians in which the clinicians experience the care modalities. Even more important, the phase-in process has allowed clinicians to observe the positive impact of alternative services used by patients in their own centers of excellence, reducing concerns about making referrals to the institute.

Involvement of Nurses at the Bedside

A key element of the ANW model is the training of nurses who provide hands-on care in alternative modalities. The support of nurses is critical to securing referrals from physicians and to educating patients about alternative care opportunities.

ENDNOTES

1. Abbott Northwestern Healthcare (ANW). 2007. "Esophageal & Gastric Care Program Supportive Services." [Online information; retrieved 4/18/07.] www.allina.com/ahs/vpci.nsf/.

2. ANW. 2005. "The Institute for Health and Healing " [Online information; retrieved 4/18/07.] www.allina.com/ahs/anw.nsf/page/ihh_home.

3. ANW (2005).

CHAPTER 5

Florida Hospital–Celebration Health: Becoming a Living Laboratory

EXECUTIVE SUMMARY

Florida Hospital–Celebration Health (FHCH) is part of the seven-facility Florida Hospital, which itself is part of a network of 17 hospitals that make up the Adventist Health System–Florida Division. FHCH was established in 1997 as part of the development of the Walt Disney Company's planned community, Celebration, located near Disney World, south of Orlando, Florida.

From its inception, FHCH has had three interrelated goals with respect to patient care. First, it desires to be a "living laboratory," providing and evaluating the latest in innovative treatments for its patients and promoting a culture of innovation among its staff. Second, it subscribes to the importance of the physical environment in promoting healing. This is reflected in the overall design of the facility and in the design of patient environments within specific units of the facility. Third, it attempts to offer a comprehensive approach to support patient health. "The difference between Celebration Health and hospitals of the past is that, while most hospitals treat only the part that has 'malfunctioned,' Celebration Health provides a total health approach which takes into account your entire way of life."[1] This is evident in the extensive array of programs available in the hospital that address lifestyle issues and promote healthy behaviors. In its mind/body/spirit approach to patient care as well as in its staff selection and training, FHCH places a strong emphasis on spirituality, reflecting its ownership by the Seventh-day Adventist Church. FHCH's goals and philosophy of care are currently being challenged by growth in demand for its services and by fiscal constraints. While innovation is still encouraged by hospital leaders, creating adequate time for managers to innovate and accumulating funds to support innovation is difficult, given the ongoing operational demands on managers' time. New program development continues to be encouraged, but often managers are expected to seek external funding sources to support it. FHCH has been able to maintain a strong spiritual dimension in relations among staff and between staff and patients, but this also requires continual affirmation of its centrality ("It's who we are") to the hospital's mission. The hospital is about to embark on an expansion of its physical facility, which will provide new opportunities for enhancing the healing environment for patients but will also test the hospital's ability to recruit new staff and physicians supportive of its faith-based approach to healing, combined with its high expectations for staff innovation.

BACKGROUND

FHCH is one of seven campuses of the Florida Hospital system, located in central Florida. The first facility in the Florida Hospital system was built in 1908 in Orlando, under the sponsorship of the Seventh-day Adventist Church, which continues to own the system. Florida Hospital now has 1,797 licensed beds and 16 walk-in urgent care centers. It intends to expand to 2,176 licensed beds by 2008. The system has 2,009 physicians on its medical staff and 4,563 nurses, of whom 3,453 work full time. It has more than a million patient visits per year and is the third largest employer in central

Florida. It offers a full range of medical services on an inpatient basis, including many high-tech specialty programs.

When FHCH was built in 1997, it intended to provide a state-of-the-art physical environment for patients that would contribute to the healing process. The hospital features architectural components that were considered at that time to be cutting edge—natural light and gardens, patient rooms designed to be family friendly, artwork, and features that dampen sound. It has about 112 beds in operation and has been at capacity for some time. There is a planned expansion to 350 beds by 2015. In addition to the usual range of services, FHCH has a cancer institute, a surgical learning institute, an Institute for Lifestyle Medicine, and a pain center.

PURSUING A PATIENT-ORIENTED STRATEGY

FHCH refers to itself as a "living laboratory" for healthcare change. It subscribes to a philosophy of "Caring for the whole person—mind, body, and spirit."[2] FHCH espouses eight principles of health, including the following:

- making healthy choices as the key to lifestyle improvement;
- the importance of the environment in the healing process;
- the desirability of being active physically, mentally, and spiritually;
- the importance of nutrition;
- the importance of interpersonal relationships, including; support of friends and family, for healing; and
- trust in God as integral to optimum health.

FHCH leaders strive to ensure that this philosophy, and its supportive principles, permeate the hospital work environment and relationships between hospital staff and patients and families. Consequently, no single individual is "in charge" of this. All hospital staff, including physicians, are expected to subscribe to a "whole person" approach to health. Those who are uncomfortable with this approach typically leave the hospital.

Culture of Innovation

FHCH attempts to promote a culture of innovation as it relates to medical technology, patient care, physical environment, and patient education. Staff members are encouraged to be innovative, with the understanding that not all innovations will be successful. Hospital leaders consistently prod managers to be innovative, asking "What's new?" and "What are you doing differently" to improve patient care. In the area of medical technology, FHCH attempts to be on the leading edge, and it has a particular emphasis on acquiring the latest imaging technology. (This can strain relations with other hospitals in the Florida Hospital system, as FHCH typically is the first hospital in the system to have access to the latest technology for imaging.) The surgical learning institute uses the latest simulation technology to train physicians, not only within the system but nationally as well.

With respect to patient care, FHCH initially adopted an innovative "universal care model." Under this model, the patient does not move from room to room within the hospital as the level of required nursing care changes. Instead, "universal units" are staffed with nurses who, collectively, have the skills and competencies to care for patients with all types of needs. This approach was supported by the hospital's physical space, with rooms designed to meet ICU size standards and equipped to handle various levels of patient acuity. Nurse-patient staffing ratios were determined by ongoing, relatively sophisticated assessments of patient acuity levels.

In theory, this should be a patient-friendly model, exposing patients to a lower risk of infection. But the model was also more challenging to staff, requiring substantial, continuing, on-site training for nurses. Early feedback on the performance of the model was promising; nurse turnover rates were relatively low and patient satisfaction was high.[3] More recently, problems arose with respect to nurse staffing and retention under the universal care model. The approach has been abandoned at FHCH primarily because ICU nurses, who consider themselves to be nurse specialists, wanted to care only for critically ill patients. Under the universal care model, FHCH found it difficult to retain ICU nurses. Recruiting and training new ICU nurses, due to higher than expected turnover rates, required substantial hospital resources. This cost, along with the potential harm to patient care caused by nurse turnover, was deemed large enough to outweigh the presumed patient benefits of the universal care model.

The hospital was designed to be an innovative physical environment that supported a mind/body/spirit approach to healing, and it received considerable attention nationally at the time it was built. Managers of units within the hospital were challenged to create welcoming physical spaces for their patients. The most notable response to this challenge occurred within the imaging services department. Typically, imaging departments are relatively stark environments, and the imaging equipment can be intimidating to patients. The unit manager at FHCH transformed the entire physical environment of the department, using a beach theme. Walls are painted with beach scenes, floors have been redone to resemble beach boardwalks, ocean sounds are played through the department's sound system, and the aroma of ocean spray permeates the area. Patients are issued beach robes in place of standard hospital gowns, sit on Adirondack chairs, and change in rooms resembling beachside cabanas. This effort has won national awards.

Softening the High-Tech Environment

Sally Grady was recruited to FHCH more than nine years ago to be part of creating something different and unique in healthcare in an organization that encouraged innovation. Although initially charged with opening a new, high-tech imaging center as a test site for the rest of the system, it was her CEO's challenge to "change the face of healthcare in imaging" that she took to heart.

How do you make the imaging experience the best that it can be?

"We came to the conclusion we wanted to do something in CT and MRI initially because that equipment can be very large and very intimidating—even to adults. People coming in specifically for MRI don't come with the idea that this is going to be a great experience. They've talked to their friends who tell them it's like being in a tomb…a dark tunnel…you'll feel claustrophobic. And MRI is not typically the first test that is ordered. It's usually one of the last, and the patient anticipates (and worries about) a definitive diagnosis. Their preconceived ideas don't help them get through the exam."

Grady and her colleagues also thought about some of the medical reasons they wanted to change the environment. They believed they could decrease the number of appointment cancellations as well as the number of adult patients who required sedation to have their MRI, which stood around 6.5 percent at that time.

"I'm a big Disney fan, and I always liked how Disney did it all when they changed the environment. From the trash cans to the signage—they attend to every minute detail to ensure the environment fit with the theme. From the time our first child was 18 months old, my husband and I would come to Disney World at least once a year. In fact, I think I was the only person who had a season ticket to Disney World before I moved here!"

Originally, Grady intended to use computer technology to create a soothing environment for patients, but she was unable to find any that was financially feasible and could be applied to a large enough area. So instead, she began to envision the three-dimensional beach theme that has made FHCH's imaging department famous.

"The beach is appealing to all ages. People love to go to the beach. They plan their vacations around it. Children love it. Adults love it. Seniors love it. Really … from age two to a hundred, there's something for everyone at the beach. So we worked with a Tampa, Florida, company to draw up some storyboards, and I was able to take those storyboards and go out and look for funding, because what I wanted to do wasn't something you're typically able to use hospital operational dollars on."

Grady secured funding partnerships with two competing companies that imaging departments do a lot of business with. They put competition aside because they believed her approach was a good thing for patients, and they both wanted to be involved.

"I really wanted to do it right. I wanted to change the flooring. I wanted to change the signage. I wanted to have what you saw, what you smelled, what you felt, what you wore remind you of being at the beach .... it really needed to affect all your senses. We wanted everything to be very nature-like and realistic. We weren't looking for murals of the tiki hut and the girl in the bikini."

"Occasionally my staff tells me I'm over the edge, but nobody ever says 'that's the dumbest thing I've ever heard.' They want to know how we can expand on it. All the high-tech equipment in the world is great, but no one has ever written me a comment card saying that my magnet was not good enough. People send you comments about the way they were treated—whether the experience was up to their expectations. It's all about how you make them feel."

As is often the case within FHCH, the unit manager was responsible for generating the funding for this innovation. To cover the costs of the renovation, contributions were secured from firms that provided the contrast material used by the imaging department. The beachside environment has been very well received by patients, and some evidence suggests that it has saved money through lower cancellation rates and reduced use of sedation. The imaging department has also created videos featuring an animated bear and a child named Max. The videos are used to educate children about the imaging experience that awaits them and allay any anxiety they might have.

Innovation in patient education occurs in a variety of ways at FHCH, supported by the principle that lifestyle management is a key to health. In 1999, Rippe Health Assessment was started as a joint venture between James M. Rippe, M.D., and FHCH, with the mission of becoming a world leader in the clinical assessment of patients' health. The assessment, which takes place over an entire day, includes a two-hour medical assessment, blood work, a nutritionist consultation, a pharmacist consultation, an exercise physiologist consultation, and radiographic studies and other diagnostics as required. Ninety-seven percent of results are available to the patient on the same day, and program staff members work with the patient to create a "road map" toward achieving individual health goals. Sixty percent of these patients return for annual or biannual assessments.

The program is limited in that it does not monitor or adjust a patient's plan over time. Patients generally are referred to their primary care providers for follow-up, which some do not find to be satisfactory. The program operates on a for-profit basis, serving primarily executives who either pay privately or have the assessment paid by their employers. Last year, the program saw between 500 and 750 new patients, but the cost is a barrier to many people. Despite a strong commitment by the hospital's leadership to find ways to support community physicians in accessing affordable lifestyle medicine resources in the hospital, the search for a viable economic model continues. The Rippe Assessment has been a cornerstone for the hospital's Institute for Lifestyle Medicine, which offers a range of diet, exercise, and educational programs to outpatients and inpatients. As with the assessment, patients pay for many of the activities out of pocket, while employers and insurance companies cover some services. Fitness center memberships are made available to hospital staff at a discounted rate as an incentive to serve as positive role models for the community, and research on the effectiveness of different lifestyle enhancement programs is an important component of the institute.

Culture of Spirituality

The influence of the Seventh-day Adventist Church in defining the hospital's mission and guiding its daily operations is significant for both staff and patients. FHCH is consistently characterized by staff as a mission-driven organization. For instance, one executive noted that FHCH is a place where it is "politically correct" to address spirituality. Staff is encouraged to pray with patients and families as part of providing care for the whole person. And patients have computerized stations at their bedsides that can be used to view spiritual videos. They are greeted with a spiritual blessing on admission and receive a blessing on discharge.

Starting from Scratch

How does a brand-new hospital, intent on creating a healing environment, build one from the ground up? Kathy Mitchell, former assistant CEO of FHCH, found herself in that position when she joined the hospital eight years ago. Now she will guide construction of a new hospital with Adventist Health in Illinois. The ground-up story started long before the history of Florida Hospital and the beginning of FHCH. It is rooted in a legacy going back to the early 1800s and Adventist Health's development of the basic principles of healthy living.

Our eight principles of health are tied into the the whole-person health approach, which in turn is threaded through all aspects of the facility's structure and operations. Treat each person as a child of God. Heal the body. Heal the spirit.

I don't believe I have it down pat. Every day I'm looking for inspiration from the Lord, and I am being inspired. I don't think you ever have it down pat. It's all about finding a way in the twenty-first century to extend the healing ministry, and how, in the new facility, do you do that? What changes will you make in the [physical] environment? How do you reflect it in every aspect of your care delivery? Where are there new opportunities to do that? And that's what's so exciting about having come from Celebration and having the opportunity to be part of the opening team of yet another new facility for Adventist Health. To do it again and know it's *not* going to be the same because there is new opportunity. There is new passion and creative energy, and there's an expectation that it'll be some new expression of our healing mission. It's electric!

A Seventh-day Adventist congregation meets at the hospital, and its pastor is involved in the hospital's pastoral care. In addition, the hospital houses a training program for chaplains. The Christian Service Committee addresses the overall spiritual environment within FHCH, and each department is responsible for developing its own Christian Service Plan. This plan typically involves a community service project undertaken by a unit outside the hospital. Each unit has funding for this activity in its budget. Another important part of the culture of spirituality in FHCH is its Spiritual Ambassador Program. Each department identifies one individual (almost always a nurse) who receives training on how to be assertive in ministering to the spiritual needs of coworkers and patients. For example, the ambassador may lead daily devotions within the unit. FHCH now has 25 ambassadors, and 17 more individuals are currently completing ambassador training.

CHALLENGES TO THE STRATEGY

FHCH has been in existence for eight years. The initial burst of enthusiasm generated by the new physical plant and ambitious administrative expectations concerning innovative leadership in patient care has now run its course. Highly publicized successes in innovation have occurred, along with some disappointments. Hospital leaders continue to expect that innovation will take place on an ongoing basis in all hospital service areas. While the organization still maintains a stated commitment to innovation in patient care directed at creating and enhancing a healing environment for patients, sustaining that commitment on a day-to-day basis is now a greater challenge than during the early years of the hospital. The planned expansion of the existing physical plant provides an opportunity to reaffirm the idea that FHCH is "different" and "cutting edge" in providing space that enhances the healing environment for patients, as well as the work environment for staff. However, expansion will create new challenges as well, particularly regarding the hospital's ability to attract the needed additional staff and managers who are comfortable with and committed to the hospital's mission and approach to patient care.

The hospital also faces the continuing challenge of attracting patients. The town of Celebration has not grown as rapidly as originally projected. Most of the patients using FHCH come from other communities in central Florida and have to pass at least one other hospital to reach FHCH. Some FHCH leaders believe the unique mission of the hospital, along with its commitment to providing a comprehensive healing environment for its patients, has been a factor in attracting patients from other communities. The concern has arisen, however, that as the hospital grows in size, it will lose some of its appeal to these patients and their families, especially if new staff are not fully committed to the hospital's approach to care.

KEYS TO SUCCESS

To date, FHCH has arguably been successful in melding innovative high-technology practices with a philosophy of treating the whole patient and a strong emphasis on spirituality in relations among staff and between staff and patients. It has remained committed to the eight principles of good health espoused by the Seventh-day Adventist Church at the same time that it has fostered a spirit of entrepreneurship among many of its staff and managers. Several factors appear to have contributed to this success.

Congruence with System Values

FHCH is part of a system of hospitals owned and managed by the Seventh-day Adventist Church. The values of the system support the mission and vision of FHCH.

Emphasis on Spirituality

Hospital leaders believe that the hospital's emphasis on the spiritual life of staff and patients has helped to attract staff with shared values that are consistent with the mission of the hospital. In general, this has resulted in FHCH being viewed as a "good place to work." Staff members who find that they are uncomfortable with the spiritual environment in the hospital typically seek employment elsewhere. Staff members who remain share a common culture and vision regarding the importance of religion in patient care at FHCH.

Ability to Secure External Funding for Innovation

To this point, managers within the hospital have been able to leverage relationships with supplier partners to attract financial support for innovative patient care modalities. In other cases, funding has been secured to support innovation through the sale of services directly to patients.

Attractiveness of the Physical Environment

The physical environment in the hospital is widely regarded as a key success factor. FHCH had the luxury of designing its physical environment from scratch, unencumbered by the limitations of an existing plant and equipment. It took advantage of this opportunity by designing a hospital that incorporated new concepts regarding how hospital spaces could be used to enhance the overall healing environment for patients. The hospital's physical plant distinguishes it from older hospitals in the area, helping to draw patients, as well as attract and retain staff.

The "Disney Connection"

The hospital is organizationally separate from the Walt Disney Company but is associated with it in public perception because of its location in the planned community of Celebration, close to Disney World. It has built on this perception internally by striving to imbue staff with the Disney culture of innovation in customer service.

ENDNOTES

1. Florida Hospital–Celebration Health. 2005. "The Story of Celebration Health." [Online information; retrieved 4/19/07.] www.celebrationhealth.com.

2. Florida Hospital–Celebration Health. 2006. "Our Mission." [Online information; retrieved 4/19/07.] celebration.smtusa.com/about/ourMission.asp.

3. Mitchell, K. 2002. "Universal Care Puts a Premium on Growth," *Nursing Spectrum* Florida Edition July 29. [Online article; retrieved 4/19/07.] community.nursingspectrum.com/MagazineArticles/article.cfm?AID=7392.

CHAPTER 6

Highline Medical Center: Maintaining the Momentum

EXECUTIVE SUMMARY

Highline Medical Center (HMC) serves an area south of downtown Seattle and has a primary campus in the city of Burien, Washington. It is an independent, not-for-profit, community organization with a variety of related entities, including inpatient facilities and a physician group. HMC describes itself as being "dedicated to cultivating a healing, pleasant, caring and nurturing environment" for its patients.[1] This philosophy has been an important part of the hospital's values since 1993, when it became the first Planetree-affiliated hospital in Washington State.

HMC views patient-centered care as its special competency and as an integral part of "who we are." As it has expanded its facilities, it has incorporated this philosophy in environmental and facility designs. It also offers a healing arts program that features a variety of services intended to support patient healing. A challenge facing HMC at present is how to maintain staff involvement in and enthusiasm for its patient-centered care philosophy and the various initiatives pertaining to it. Because this approach has been part of the hospital for some time and the hospital has attempted to embed it in day-to-day patient care, it is not as visible to staff and leadership as it was in its early years. Staff turnover, although relatively low, reinforces this challenge.

Currently, HMC is engaged in an organization-wide effort to improve patient satisfaction. This effort has refocused attention on the hospital's historical commitment to a Planetree approach, but it has also raised questions about how to reinvigorate that approach so that it reinforces new HMC initiatives to improve patient satisfaction scores. HMC leadership has no intention of altering HMC's values or its commitment to a holistic approach to patient care. But there is a sense that, even after 13 years, the potential of this approach has yet to be fully realized within HMC.

BACKGROUND

HMC began as Burien General Hospital in 1958, changing its name to Highline Community Hospital in 1978 when it became a community, not-for-profit facility. Its physical plant has grown steadily over time, beginning with a five-story addition in 1985. The hospital purchased Riverton General Hospital, located about four miles away, in 1989. This facility, renamed the Specialty Center, contains programs relating to restorative care/skilled nursing care, geriatric psychiatric care, acute rehabilitation, chemical dependency treatment, home health care, physical and respiratory therapy, emergency services, and radiology. As of 2004, the hospital as a whole is licensed to operate 269 beds; 106 acute beds are in operation at the main campus and 70 at the Specialty Center campus. In 1998, the hospital added a new wing containing a childbirth center, a medical/oncology unit, a community health education center, and exercise facilities for cardiac rehabilitation patients. When the hospital opened a new cancer center in 2005, it changed its name to Highline Medical Center to reflect the broad scope of services it provides. The Highline Medical Group was formed in 1990 as a subsidiary of HMC and now has 19 clinics and 50 physicians. HMC also owns interests in medical office buildings, a sleep disorder center, an imaging practice, and a physical therapy group. It has contractual agreements with Swedish Medical Center in Seattle for radiation therapy and selected cardiac services.

Approximately 1,250 employees work at HMC, and 250 to 300 physicians are on its medical staff, almost all of whom are board certified. In 2004, 20 physicians admitted approximately 46 percent of HMC's patients. About 37 percent of admissions originate in the hospital's primary service area. It has a 20 percent market share, based on combined admissions from its primary and secondary service areas, which have a total population of slightly less than 400,000. HMC's service area has an aging, ethnically diverse population, and population growth has been relatively slow. The area is home to people of 80 distinct nationalities, and 60 to 70 different languages are spoken by children in the local school districts. The potential for service area expansion is limited by geography and by the location of competitors. HMC's major competitors for inpatient services are the large tertiary referral centers in central Seattle.

About 42 percent of HMC's gross patient revenues are from Medicare patients, 17 percent from Medicaid, and 31 percent from private insurance. HMC has a greater percentage of charity care than most of its competitors. Nevertheless, HMC is relatively stable financially, showing improvement in its profit margin from 3 percent to 5 percent over the last five years. It is now planning to upgrade the older parts of its main campus facility, add new patient rooms, and increase its emergency department capabilities. In September 2004, it embarked on a major, systemwide effort to improve its patient satisfaction scores. It found that, when benchmarked against other hospitals, its scores were not competitive.

PURSUING A PATIENT-ORIENTED STRATEGY

In 1992, three members of the hospital's administrative staff attended a conference where a presentation was given about Planetree. They returned enthusiastic about the potential for the

Planetree philosophy to improve nurse morale at the Specialty Center. They felt that Planetree's emphasis on family involvement in care was particularly appropriate for the type of services provided at the Specialty Center, especially rehabilitation, geriatric psychiatry, and behavioral health. They were also interested in incorporating a healing arts approach in the treatment of these patients, including pet therapy, art therapy, and music therapy. Most importantly, the hospital leaders felt that Planetree was a good fit for what they had been trying to accomplish more generally. It was a way to "name what we do."

Reconfiguring Hospital Spaces

The physical environment of a hospital can represent a visual commitment to a patient-centered philosophy and is one factor that can influence both staff and patient satisfaction. Mark Benedum, chief operating officer of HMC, notes, "In almost every hospital there's an old section and a newer section. We thought it would be creative to incorporate the Planetree philosophy by naming our wings after trees. But staff continues to think of them as 'the new wing' and 'the old wing.'

"The older wing at Highline was built 25 years ago at a time when the hospital was 'stretching' to build the building. The patient rooms are primarily semiprivate and the nursing units are particularly tight in support areas. Interestingly, the design was based on a triangle and, as a result, central work areas are not as large as they would be using a rectangular design. There's just not enough core space to accommodate the increased amount of equipment that has been added over the years. So when we look at the combination of the staff, the congestion, and the lack of storage space, the two wings are entirely different physical environments. Then you lay Planetree philosophy on top of that— open visitation and encouraging families to take part in the patients' care in semiprivate rooms ... it can get overwhelming.

We have always believed that the physical environment is a big influence, but hadn't really thought how deeply it could impact many aspects of patient care delivery, including clinical quality. For example, we know of hospitals that documented their infection rates dropping when they went to all-private rooms."

But how does physical environment affect patient and staff satisfaction scores? When Benedum and colleagues found significant differences in Press Ganey patient satisfaction scores between their older and newer wings, it caused them to take a closer look at staff satisfaction. Expecting to find higher scores correlated with the new wing, they were surprised to find mixed results. While space and privacy seem to be important to patients, the relational environment may be more important to staff than the physical environment. "In fact," says Benedum, "the nursing staff from one of the units in the older wing that works under the most difficult physical conditions rated their work environment as high as the newer units. Knowing what we know about the leadership, communication, and decision making on these units, I am realizing that staff satisfaction may be more closely related to how they feel about their supervisor."

HMC, however, continues to address satisfaction scores from both fronts. Grace Henley, director of human resources, notes that on the newer units, "there is often a 'pride of ownership'" that translates into staff taking better care of their workspace, thus easing the cost of routine wear and tear. The newer areas of that facility also have more available spaces for staff. "In the older wing, we have gone in and done some refurbishing and a little bit of remodeling to upgrade the look and modernize the space, even though we weren't able to go to private rooms and create the same kind of spaces as the new areas. I think this has made a difference from a staff perspective. Now staff members don't feel as though they have to apologize for the rooms, and they feel better about the care they give because they are not working in 'substandard space' anymore."

In moving ahead with a new capital expansion plan, converting semiprivate rooms into private rooms remains a priority in Benedum's mind. "At each of our staff communication forums, I asked attendees how they would feel about having a roommate during a hospital stay, and the consensus always favors privacy. I think it's pretty ingrained in our culture now, and especially among healthcare providers, that [patients] don't want a roommate when they enter the hospital, and they would rather deliver care to patients in private rooms."

They had been discussing the need to develop a distinctive competency for the hospital, but they knew they could not "out-tech" or "out-buy" their large, tertiary hospital competitors. Some of the executives visited Mid Columbia Hospital in The Dalles, Oregon, which had implemented a similar approach, and their visit solidified their support for the Planetree model.

Initially, they took a "soft" approach to introducing the model by implementing initiatives at the Specialty Center alone. Within two years, the administrative team decided to expand the initiative to include both the Specialty Center and HMC's main campus. At this time, they hired both a Planetree program manager and a Planetree facilitator. The hospital then committed to broad-based training of staff in Planetree principles. An off-site training program for all 1,250 hospital staff members was held, and people were trained in groups of 25 members. HMC encountered resistance on the part of some staff, but they expected this would "go away." However, there was also "excitement, enthusiasm and some confusion," as no one knew exactly where the hospital would end up in its attempt to incorporate Planetree principles into its vision and everyday operations. Shortly after, a healing arts program was established on the Specialty Center campus. This program has grown to offer a variety of services, including music, art, clinically based aromatherapy, massage, meditation, patient comfort touch, and pet therapy.

As part of its Planetree program, HMC opened a Planetree health library at its main campus, located next to the hospital's cafeteria and gift shop and overlooking a healing garden. The library offers an array of materials and information sources for patients, and it is used by staff as well. While the library was a highly visible symbol of the hospital's commitment to Planetree, the implementation of the Planetree philosophy at HMC took another major step forward with the opening of a new hospital wing (the Cedar Wing) in 1998. This wing incorporated family kitchens, larger patient rooms, water details, artwork, and other architectural features designed to make patients feel at home and to relieve patient and family stress. In combination with staff training, it illustrated the full potential of a patient-centered approach to healing. It also moved this approach onto the main campus in a significant way. Now, new staff receive training in the Planetree philosophy and HMC's values with respect to patient-centered care as part of their orientation. But a continuing challenge for hospital administration is how to make the Planetree approach and initiatives part of the fabric of the hospital, and not just something the hospital staff views as "one more thing to do."

The hospital employs a Planetree coordinator and a Planetree librarian, and both positions are funded as part of the overall hospital budget. The healing arts facilitator, who has been funded by the hospital and through patient revenues since 1993, is combined with the manager of marketing position at the Specialty Center. The foundation and the hospital's volunteer organization have funded some of the Planetree projects. The guiding management philosophy with respect to Planetree is to structure programs relating to patient care so that they are "owned" at the unit level, with support provided by the coordinator. Manuals are developed centrally for teaching different patient care programs in the units, but units bear the expense of "purchasing" these educational resources and finding time to train staff. They build these expenses into their budgets. Unit leaders are expected to report on progress or activities at regularly scheduled administrative meetings, but they are not held to specific, detailed performance objectives.

CHALLENGES TO THE STRATEGY

Obtaining nurse buy-in for various Planetree initiatives is an ongoing challenge, and time and effort are required to bring them along and gain their support. Often, nurses see these initiatives as competing for their time and attention with other hospital programs aimed at improving quality of care. However, hospital leaders point to a decline in staff turnover from 25 percent in 2000 to 13 percent in 2005 and believe that the hospital's patient-centered approach, built around Planetree, has been a factor in this trend, as well as an important staff recruiting tool for the hospital. However, from 2002 to 2005, the administration's attention to Planetree initiatives and their implementation waned somewhat, as indicated by less regular reporting at administrative meetings; more recently, the administrative initiative to improve patient satisfaction scores in the hospital has focused new attention on how Planetree efforts have been received by patients. While HMC's patient satisfaction scores are relatively high, they did not meet the expectations of the hospital's administration. Scores were highest (in the 85th to the 97th percentile) for patients treated in the new hospital wing, where there are private rooms, more amenities, a lower ambient noise level, and open nursing stations; the scores were much lower for patients treated in the older parts of the facility.

With respect to the healing arts program, acceptance and support on the part of clinicians has increased over time, with a new impetus provided by the opening of the hospital's cancer center. Some effort has been made to integrate selected healing arts therapies with bedside care. For example, therapeutic touch training for nurses is available, as is training in aromatherapy. With respect to other services, physicians must write "prescriptions" for a service to be delivered in the inpatient setting. The healing arts program then arranges for a therapist to respond to the physician's order. These therapists are not credentialed through the hospital; most are independent practitioners who are affiliated with the hospital.

While the number of physicians who regularly initiate orders for complementary/alternative medicine therapies for their patients is limited, most physicians in the Highline Medical Group are open to writing orders in response to patient requests. At the cancer center, use of these therapies for outpatient pain management has been much in demand. HMC's younger hospitalists could be open to the greater use of alternative therapies for hospitalized patients. However, to date no formal program has been directed at educating them about the healing arts services.

Since the initiation of the Planetree efforts, no one physician has accepted the responsibility for championing them. Physicians have been slow to use alternative therapies in their practices, but they also have not expressed overt opposition to them. These therapies and their availability "fly under the radar" for most of the medical staff. The one exception occurred when aromatherapy was initially introduced. Some physicians opposed it because it appeared that the manner in which the therapy was being used did not have a clear clinical foundation.

Funding for the Planetree efforts at HMC comes from a variety of sources. The salaries of the coordinator and the librarian are line items in the hospital's budget. Outpatient therapies are sometimes reimbursed by third-party payers, but inpatient therapy is not. There are relatively few costs for the inpatient Planetree programs beyond personnel. Volunteer time and donations are an important additional source of financial support; hospital volunteers have raised and donated about $75,000 per year to "patient comfort"–related programs. The Planetree effort, to date, has not been required to demonstrate a positive return on investment. Hospital leaders doubt that it would be possible to attribute increased patient revenues, or reduced hospital costs, directly to Planetree programs or activities. However, they remain supportive of the patient-centered care philosophy, although some think the time is ripe for a refocusing of the model to support improvements in patient satisfaction.

Renewing the Commitment

Paul Tucker, CEO of HMC suggests that keeping the Planetree philosophy fresh beyond the honeymoon phase, despite competing priorities, is not difficult when it is congruent with who you are as an organization and who you are as an individual.

In the beginning, we chose to become a Planetree affiliate because it was a way to attach a name to our culture, to the way we already treated people. It said to the world, "This is who we are."

For the past year and a half, we have been looking at how we are meeting (or aren't meeting) the emotional needs of our patients as reflected by our Press Ganey satisfaction scores. We asked the committee to help us interpret the satisfaction scores and propose initiatives to address patient expectations in this area. One of the suggestions they came up with was "scripting."

Now, to some people, scripting seems phony. I suppose it can be phony if you aren't careful, but it can also be a really good strategy. I learned about the value of scripting when I purchased my last cell phone. One day, while I was at my sons' track meet, I was passing time by trying to figure out a few of the cell phone functions without referring to the user's guide. Being as compulsive as I am, I kept pushing keys even when the phone warned me to stop. As a result, I managed to shut it down completely and needed to call the cell phone distributor for directions on how to get it up and running again, which they provided. At the end of the call, they said, "Mr. Tucker, before we hang up, is there anything else we can do for you today?" and I thought, "Gee, that's nice." Unfortunately, I started playing with the phone again the next day, and shut it down again. In fact, I managed to shut it down completely four or five times over a period of days. Each time I called the distributor, I talked to a different person. And each time, the person ended our conversation by asking the same question, "Is there anything else I can do for you before we hang up?"

Now obviously, by the second time around, I realized that the question was part of each employee's "script," and it was something they were supposed to say. It was not necessarily people being spontaneously nice to me. But I realized that it made me feel good each time they said it. I didn't care that it was scripted. I got the message that they were concerned about me and willing to do something for me if I asked. This was a powerful experience.

When I go into orientation every month, I tell this story to our new staff. I tell them that scripting is simply a reminder about "the right thing to say." Whether it's me, a nurse, a dietitian, a kitchen delivery person, or a housekeeper interacting with the patient, we can all be responsive to the patient's emotional needs and sensitive to the many inconveniences of being in hospital. For example, a patient's blood test may be delayed by an hour, which means they can't eat until the blood test is done, even if they are very hungry. We need to let them know we feel a little bit of their pain and give them enough information that they can understand the delay. I think this type of awareness is an outgrowth of our Planetree philosophy over time and an example of how we keep it alive on a day-to-day basis.

KEYS TO SUCCESS

HMC has more than a decade of experience implementing a hospital-wide approach to patient-centered care using the Planetree model. HMC executives believe several factors have been influential in its success to date.

Sustained Support from Hospital Administration

From the beginning, HMC leadership has supported the concept of patient-centered care and made it central to the hospital's culture. It has communicated consistently and clearly that "This is who we are."

Gradual Implementation

After an initial hospital-wide educational effort, patient-centered programs have been implemented in different ways in various parts of the hospital, taking advantage of other developments, such as the construction of the Cedar Wing and the opening of the new cancer center. The latter provided the opportunity to integrate complementary services such as naturopathy and acupuncture into care, due to the support of the oncologists in the center. Over time, leaders have increasingly recognized that staff preparation must take place to the point that they are accepting of a new service or program. Proceeding before staff support has been established reduces the likelihood of success.

Recognizing Financial Limitations

Although HMC is a financially stable hospital, it has limited funds to allocate to programmatic efforts. The patient-centered care initiatives have been scaled to accommodate this financial reality and have relied considerably on volunteer fund-raising for support.

Taking Advantage of New Construction

When HMC has undertaken new construction, it has incorporated design principles advocated by Planetree. Designing new spaces that support patient-centered care efforts has contributed to improved nurse satisfaction.

ENDNOTE

1. Highline Medical Center (HMC). 2007. "Hospital Highlights." [Online information; retrieved 4/19/07.] highlinemedicalcenter.org/about/index.php

CHAPTER 7

St. Charles Medical Center–Bend: Adjusting to Change

EXECUTIVE SUMMARY

The St. Charles Medical Center facility in Bend, Oregon (SCMCB), is a not-for-profit, community hospital providing a complete range of services to residents of central and eastern Oregon. Historically, the hospital has had a strong culture of patient-centered care. This culture was reaffirmed in the early 1990s through an initiative termed Healing Health Care (HHC). HHC focuses on patients and families as well as hospital staff members. The hospital is known nationally for its holistic care, the healing designs of its facilities, and innovative programs such as 24-hour "total room service" for patients. Recent additions to the hospital plant have continued to incorporate design components that support HHC. A new CEO, who joined the organization two years ago, was perceived by some staff as shifting the hospital's emphasis from HHC to financial performance and expansion. The CEO recently left the organization, but his tenure created some uncertainty about the organization's longer-term commitment to HHC. In part because of nurse concerns about a perceived weakening of administrative support for HHC, the hospital narrowly avoided what one executive termed a "nurse meltdown" at the end of 2005.

Throughout this period, nurses and medical staff have been involved in a facility-wide implementation of a new $14 million EMR system, which the CEO who recently left characterized as "one of the biggest changes we've implemented in the history of our organization" and which some staff felt intruded on the maintenance of an HHC approach in relations with patients. In the face of these challenges, an important question for SCMCB now concerns the centrality of HHC to its mission going forward and, if that centrality is reaffirmed, the implications for staff and patients.

BACKGROUND

Cascade Healthcare Community owns two facilities, SCMCB and St. Charles Medical Center–Redmond (both in central Oregon), and it manages two other hospitals. The hospital in Bend has 216 beds (after an expansion in 2004) and 2,000 employees. The Redmond facility is much smaller, with about 400 employees. SCMCB offers a full range of services, with the exception of transplant surgery and major burn care. Many of these services, such as open heart surgery, neurosurgery, comprehensive cancer care, inpatient rehabilitation for stroke and major injuries, and sophisticated imaging technologies, are typically found only in larger metropolitan facilities. SCMCB is Oregon's only Level II trauma center east of the Cascade Mountains, and it has the area's only Level III neonatal ICU. Its Healing Health Campus, which includes a residential mental health treatment facility and an apartment complex for patients with persistent mental illness, is located next to SCMCB, and the region's primary medical air ambulance service is based at SCMCB as well.

This broad scope of services reflects SCMCB's role as the major regional referral center in eastern Oregon, serving about 230,000 people in a 32,000 square mile area (larger than the geographic area of Vermont, Connecticut, Massachusetts, Delaware, and New

Hampshire combined). SCMCB has frequently been listed among the best hospitals in the nation for heart, cancer, orthopedic, and neurosurgical care, and it is ranked among the 100 top U.S. hospitals for overall quality of care and operational efficiency.

The population in the area served by the Bend and Redmond facilities of SCMC is growing rapidly. New physicians and caregivers have moved to the area to serve its expanding population. As a result, 65 to 70 percent of community physicians and more than 50 percent of other caregivers are new in the past five to seven years. The population growth has strained the capacity of the two facilities. Consequently, facility expansion is now underway. In Bend, the hospital added 46 inpatient rooms in late 2004 and early 2005. In 2004, it completed a new medical diagnostics unit. In 2005, it opened an orthopedic and neurosurgical medical office building and outpatient surgery center (a joint venture with physicians). Between 2003 and 2006, SCMCB doubled the size of its emergency department and added psychiatric hold rooms. A new heart center (another joint venture with physicians) opened in fall 2006. It also opened a new outpatient pharmacy, expanded its imaging space, and had plans to break ground for an expansion of its Family Birthing Center in 2006. Inpatient capacity is being reconfigured at the Redmond facility to provide private patient rooms, improve the healing environment, and ultimately relieve some of the pressures on SCMCB with the planned expansion of surgical facilities.

In total, the costs of these new projects, including facilities, technology, and equipment, will be in excess of $128 million, causing SCMC to take on considerable new debt. This is seen as feasible because the debt load of the hospital has historically been quite low. The hospital generated a 3 percent margin on operations this past year. At Bend, 42 percent of hospital charges are for Medicare patients, 32 percent for managed care, 8 percent for commercial insurance, and 10 percent for Medicaid.

SCMCB competes with some hospitals west of the Cascade Mountains, as well as hospitals in Boise, Idaho, in some specialty service lines at the outer fringes of its service area. Basically, however, its geographic location protects it from competition with other inpatient facilities, resulting in about a 95 percent inpatient market share in some service lines. At present, the primary competition for SCMCB is from physicians on its medical staff. Three physician-owned ambulatory surgery centers are operating in Bend and Redmond, and SCMCB partnered with some of its own physicians (effectively splitting the revenue) to build an ambulatory surgery center for outpatient orthopedic surgery. There are also eight MRI machines in Bend; three are owned through hospital/physician partnerships, and five are independently owned. SCMCB forecasts that competition with its medical staff, just on the basis of imaging services, will subtract $1.5 million from its bottom line in 2007.

In 2006, SCMC was in a state of flux. Staff felt the pressures created by ongoing acclimatization to the new EMR system, which went live on October 12, 2005, after two years of testing and planning. Construction was occurring at both Bend and Redmond, and there was a competitive climate between the hospital and the medical staff. Then, SCMC's CEO took administrative leave in February 2006 and left the organization in March. This created uncertainty among staff concerning the future direction for the hospital in general, and for HHC in particular. Some of this angst was addressed with the board's appointment of an internal candidate—a system vice president and former executive of the Redmond hospital—as the new CEO in May 2006.

Complicating this picture further, relations between hospital nurses and administration were tense, although some reconciliation of differences now seems to be occurring. SCMCB employs 600 nurses, and the Redmond facility has 200. While 95 percent are permanent staff, 50 percent are part-time employees, reflecting lifestyle choices common to the region. All belong to a union, and turnover of nursing staff has been only 5 percent to 10 percent per year. In the last two years, patient satisfaction measures have lagged behind SCMCB's traditional 90th percentile rankings.

In late 2005, the nurses at SCMCB rebelled against what they perceived to be organizational changes undertaken without appropriate consultation. Some nurses felt that these changes were having a negative impact on patient care. After much discussion, a "letter of intent" was signed between nurses and administration that committed each group to work together to rebuild their relationship.

PURSUING A PATIENT-ORIENTED STRATEGY

The hospital in Bend was established in 1918 by the Sisters of St. Joseph of Tipton, Indiana, a Catholic order. In the early 1970s, St. Charles Medical Center, Inc., was created, ending ownership ties with the order. The Sisters donated existing hospital assets to the new not-for-profit corporation and turned over hospital governance to a local board of directors, though the Sisters retained board membership and the presidency of the hospital.

A major new facility was opened in 1975 with the goal of providing all needed medical services for citizens of Oregon residing east of the Cascade Mountains. It was the administration's vision that care at this facility should address the mind/body/spiritual needs of all patients. In 1990, the hospital embarked on a patient-centered restructuring to prepare for managed care and a rapidly changing healthcare environment. A task force, including employees and physicians, was charged to develop the mission enhancement plan. The work of this task force became the HHC philosophy, which "is based on the belief that the essence of healing is our relationships with the people we serve and that nearly everything in the environment has an effect on recovery and well being, either enhancing or impairing the healing process. With the overriding goal of 'healing ourselves, our relationships, and our community,' Healing Health Care is about our intention to assure [sic] that all factors in the hospital environment enhance opportunities for healing—combining both the science and the art of care."[1] Leaders of SCMCB say that HHC is "not a program—it is the way we do business," that it is "organic," and that, consequently, people "feel something different" when they enter the hospital. The HHC approach is manifested in a variety of ways within SCMCB, as illustrated by the following examples.

Relationship-Centered Care

The goal of relationship-centered care is for the caregiver and patient to be in a relationship that promotes healing. For instance, the nurse may sit with the patient, hear his story, and demonstrate an interest in the patient as a whole person, not just a disease or problem to be addressed. The caregiver is expected to be "present" with the patient, referring to the philosophy of "therapeutic presence." To support this concept, over the past two years clinicians have focused on primary care nursing, with a nurse responsible for a therapeutic relationship and plan of care throughout the patient's hospital stay.

Health Coach

A health coach is available to help patients create a personalized health enhancement plan that emphasizes a holistic approach to wellness.

Health Resource Center

The Health Resource Center "is dedicated to helping patients, families and community members find the resources and information they need to make informed decisions about their health."[2] It consists of a free public lending library containing clinical textbooks and journals; health information packets;

online access; support groups; some complementary services such as massage therapy, yoga, and relaxation methods; and the Health and Care Store. The center has been very well received by patients and the community as a whole but does not bring in enough revenue to sustain itself financially. Its shortfalls are subsidized by the hospital.

Guest Services Host Program

The Guest Services Host Program was initiated in September 2005 with funding provided by a grant from the St. Charles Foundation. Each person coming through the door of SCMCB is met by a host who can answer questions and help put the visitor at ease. Although in its infancy, the program has been received enthusiastically by the community.

Caregiver Assistance Program

Confidential counseling is available at the hospital for caregivers and family members, including referral as necessary to resources outside of the hospital.

People-Centered Teams

Hospital-based caregivers receive two and one-half days of training in teamwork skills, including communication tools, so that they can function more effectively as teams in caring for patients. All caregivers are required to complete this training in their first year of employment, and the cost of training is charged to each department's budget. Previously, caregivers were required to be retrained every five years, but this has been dropped. The effective use of people-centered team skills is assessed as part of caregivers' performance reviews.

Environmental Design

SCMCB has attempted to make the physical environment in the hospital conducive to patient healing and supportive of caregivers in being a therapeutic presence. For example, walls and floors are decorated in warm tones, art is commonplace, volunteers regularly play the grand piano located in the hospital's lobby, and televisions in patient rooms default to channels with nature scenes, relaxing music, and guided imagery. In the newly constructed tower, rooms are large enough to accommodate major pieces of equipment, caregivers, and family members all at once. The rooms have large windows with expansive views, built-in sleep couches, private bathrooms, and desks with data ports for computer access.

Food Service

SCMCB is known nationally for its innovative 24-hour total room service program for patients. Patients are able to order meals or snacks (within dietary guidelines) at any time, and delivery occurs within 20 to 30 minutes. The hospital believes this approach promotes patient healing by giving patients an additional measure of control in their hospital stay. Although it would seem to be expensive, the hospital has found that it is cost-neutral or even less expensive than traditional hospital food services because of avoided food waste.

Complementary Therapies

Every nurse is trained to provide relaxation therapy and guided imagery, and some are also trained in therapeutic touch. Aromatherapy is also offered in some units of the hospital. These services are regarded as part of nursing practice and can be carried out without a physician order. Therapeutic touch was controversial when it was first offered and segments within the local religious community picketed the facility (the facility, in turn, explained the principle of therapeutic touch and waited out the protest). Other therapies are available to patients on request. In a policy that began two years ago, each unit within the hospital has a designated HHC resource person. This person is responsible for staff competency in relaxation therapy—therapeutic touch is not a required core competency for nurses. In general, physicians are accepting of nurses developing healing relationships with patients and regard pet therapy and massage therapy as innocuous. However, they are reported to be more skeptical of therapeutic touch and somewhat resistant to other therapies. With ongoing population growth in the area, more providers of complementary therapies are establishing practices in Bend and Redmond, and this could ultimately increase the demand for these services on the part of hospital patients.

Hospital administration does not regard the ongoing programs that support its HHC approach to be of major financial significance. Many of the costs are built into department budgets and, in some cases, patients reimburse the hospital for the services they receive (e.g., massage therapy). Many patient-oriented activities are subsidized through funding provided by the St. Charles Foundation. And the hospital board and leadership continue to stress their commitment to HHC principles. However, recent events within the hospital are causing leadership to revisit how to carry out HHC more effectively in the future.

Rethinking Hospital Food Services

"When you think of fine cuisine, 'hospital food' is not the first phrase that comes to mind. In fact, it might be the last. So in the mid-1990s when St. Charles Medical Center–Bend, Oregon, wanted to improve quality and service for patient meals, we didn't look to other hospitals to set the standard. Why strive to be the best among a field of poor performers?"

Todd Sprague, corporate communications manager for SCMCB at the time this book was written, discussed the organization's goal to raise the bar for food service.

As a starter, we decided to send some of our key staff to the Ritz-Carlton for a site visit. While we were also expanding and redesigning our kitchens and public cafeterias, in what turned out to be an award-winning design, we wanted to tackle some of the key challenges related to patient meals.

Like most hospitals at the time—and even today—regular meals (breakfast, lunch, and dinner) were handled through a system in which patients were required to select items they thought they would like to eat the next day (ordering 24 hours in advance) from a very limited menu. Meals were then prepared en masse in a tray-line system and hauled to the patient care areas on a schedule that hinged on the convenience of the hospital, not the patient.

While we knew that the approach to regular meals left much to be desired, our first foray into room service was aimed at improving between-meal service. Traditionally, between-meal needs (patients returning from surgery late in the day or getting hungry in the middle of the night) were handled by stocking significant amounts of sandwiches, gelatin, crackers, and beverages in patient care areas. This system resulted in a lot of waste or loss (food spoilage, food being shared with families, staff members grabbing an occasional snack, etc.).

By building in some of our service lessons from the Ritz-Carlton, reconfiguring our staffing, and making some changes in processes and facilities, we were able to remove most food from the patient care areas, offer a larger menu to patients for between-meal snacks, and provide on-demand room service between meals with a 20-to-30 minute response time (better than most hotels) and a built-in review process to ensure compliance with dietary restrictions.

The result? Patient satisfaction increased and we actually saved about $30,000 per year. We also improved caregiver access to meals on the evening and night shifts.

After a few years of positive experience with 'partial' room service, we took a hard look at the possibility of expanding to total room service for patient meals. It was becoming difficult to maintain two approaches to food service. We soon confirmed that patients who order food a day in advance often select items they are not hungry for the next day when the food actually arrives. That translated into two pounds of food waste per patient per day.

Seizing that opportunity, we made some additional changes to staffing and facilities; greatly expanded the menu (with an emphasis on cooking from scratch); widened the time window for breakfast, lunch, and dinner to give patients more control over their eating times; and retained a menu of items available 24 hours a day for between-meal snacks.

With the implementation of total room service in 1999, food waste dropped to nearly zero, and patient satisfaction soared to the 99th percentile. Costs remained pretty much the same (eliminating food waste balanced out staffing and other expenses related to total room service). We later implemented the same type of system at St. Charles Medical Center–Redmond, our 48-bed community hospital, with similar success.

While food service is not highly correlated with overall patient satisfaction, it does offer patients a measure of control in an otherwise unfamiliar environment. Food also plays an important role in the physical and emotional health of the patient. Paying attention to food, especially in a way that improved quality without increasing costs, fit perfectly within our "Healing Health Care" philosophy. In our relationship-focused organization—with its emphasis on body, mind and spirit—total room service was the right thing to do for all the right reasons.

CHALLENGES TO THE STRATEGY

The nursing staff at SCMCB plays a critical role in implementing the HHC philosophy at the hospital. Over the past decade, SCMCB has attracted nurses who are comfortable with this approach, and nurse turnover has been low. But in the past two years, some nurses have questioned the degree to which the hospital continues to support the HHC philosophy. The implementation of the EMR system has provided a focal point for the frustration of some nurses, who say, in essence, "It's hard to personalize care while pulling around a computer." Nurses have had difficulty addressing the new demands of the system while maintaining a therapeutic relationship with patients. In addition to EMR system implementation issues, some nurses believe that facility expansion and financial issues have distracted hospital leadership from HHC and that the recent hospital CEO never fully understood or was committed to HHC.

There is a strong sense among hospital leaders that the recent confrontation with SCMCB nurses has changed the environment within the hospital and called into question the future of HHC. At the least, both the leadership and the nursing staff recognize the need to rebuild mutual trust, with a renewed, shared understanding of the future role of HHC in the hospital, which is central in this regard. The hospital was under interim leadership for a period, but its new CEO was selected in part due to his perceived relationship-building skills. Moving forward, the new CEO and the executive team will attempt to reaffirm HHC as a fundamental element of care at SCMCB. For example, they have initiated a program titled Pathfinder Project: Revisiting Our Organization's Soul, whereby specially trained caregivers are engaging others throughout the organization in discussions to reintroduce the mission, values, and HHC philosophy.

Hospital leadership is also focusing attention on improving relationships with its physician staff, in light of the increasing competitive tensions between physicians and the hospital. This effort may assume the highest priority, absorbing administrative time and attention. Another factor affecting SCMCB's ability to pursue patient-centered care is that many new physicians on the medical staff do not view reaffirming the role of HHC as a critical issue for the hospital. Hospital leadership has observed that it could have done a better job, over the years, of educating new physicians about HHC and its importance to the hospital as a guiding philosophy.

In addressing these challenges, SCMCB can draw on a strong reservoir of support for HHC within both the hospital and the community. SCMCB has not attempted to measure HHC's impact on the hospital. Technically, this would be very difficult to accomplish. Despite this, HHC has become such an important force in defining the hospital's culture that its values now appear to be accepted at all levels within the organization. As one caregiver noted, "It's the right thing to do, it's what patients want, and it's what we want for ourselves and our families." Hospital leadership has observed that, because HHC has been so deeply embedded in the hospital for such a long time, the hospital may have "let its guard down." Addressing the present challenges can provide an opportunity to reinvigorate SCMCB's commitment to the HHC philosophy within the organization.

KEYS TO SUCCESS

The challenges now facing SCMCB in maintaining its HHC philosophy and practice should not obscure the success that it has experienced for more than a decade in this area. This success can be explained by several considerations.

Visionary Leadership

Since the mid-1970s, SCMCB has had leaders with a strong vision for patient-centered care and the ability to articulate that vision to audiences internal and external to the hospital. The consistency of their vision, and their ability to mobilize support for it, are important in explaining the hospital's success.

Supportive External Environment

Until recently, SCMCB has operated with relatively limited competition. This has allowed hospital leadership to focus more time and attention on HHC than might have occurred in a more competitive market.

Caregiver Buy-In

The HHC approach features a central role for caregivers, especially nurses. Generally, nurses have appreciated their expanded caregiving role at the patient's bedside and have been supportive of HHC as a result. Staff turnover has been low and patient satisfaction is high.

Sustained Innovation

On a regular basis, SCMCB reassesses the resources and training necessary to support an HHC philosophy of care. It has put new programs in place relating both to staff training and patient support to meet needs or address problems as they have arisen.

Strategic Focus

The hospital's healing philosophy has been linked to its strategic plan, mission, and vision. Hospital leaders have seen it as an important strategic initiative and have established clear lines of responsibility, accountability, and authority.

Tenacity

Implementing a healing philosophy challenges the status quo and requires a change of mental model for all concerned. As a result, many challenges to the concepts, practices, and initiatives have arisen. Implementation takes time, and hospital leaders believe that tenacity in pursuit of the HHC philosophy over time has been a key to success.

Design of New Physical Space

As SCMCB has expanded, it has used that opportunity to design physical space that supports its HHC philosophy. This commitment has solidified support for HHC within the hospital and in the community.

ENDNOTES

1. Patient Centered Teams. 2004. Unpublished internal document.

2. St. Charles Medical Center. 2006. "Health Resource Center." [Online information; retrieved 4/18/06.] www.scmc.org/services_HealthResourceCenter.html.

CHAPTER 8

North Hawaii Community Hospital: A Blended Medicine Perspective

EXECUTIVE SUMMARY

North Hawaii Community Hospital (NHCH) was built in 1996 as a model for "blended medicine," where the best in traditional and nontraditional approaches to treatment would be available to patients. It describes itself as offering "a full spectrum of acute care hospital services with a commitment to patient-centered care that treats the patient as a whole person—mind, body, and spirit—in the context of family, culture and community. Designed as a 'healing instrument,' NHCH is fast becoming a prototype for the careful integration of select complementary healing practices with high quality medical care."[1]

In its design and philosophy of care, NHCH has attempted to incorporate elements of the culture of Hawaii. It has received substantial financial support from philanthropy; donations from Earl Bakken, former CEO of a large, medical-device manufacturer, were especially important in constructing the hospital. His leadership was also a key factor in developing the hospital's blended medicine approach. While NHCH has received national attention for its building and its patient care philosophy, a strong feeling among staff prevails that it has not yet fulfilled its promise and potential. NHCH has been limited in this respect by its relatively small size and its ongoing financial challenges. On a year-to-year basis, NHCH typically loses money on operations, making up the shortfall through philanthropy. This restricts the hospital's ability to pursue new initiatives directed at enhancing its healing environment and makes it difficult for the hospital to sustain existing efforts without external support.

BACKGROUND

NHCH, located in Waimea on the Big Island of Hawaii, opened in 1996. Since its inception, the hospital has been managed by Adventist Health, a not-for-profit company headquartered in Roseville, California, that manages 20 hospitals and 16 home health agencies in four western states (Hawaii, California, Oregon, and Washington). NHCH has 40 acute care beds, serves a population of 35,000 residents in a catchment area of approximately 1,000 square miles, and has limited competition from other hospitals. NHCH has 144 physicians on staff, 464 employees, and 75 volunteers. Approximately 175 nurses work at NHCH, and staff turnover is about 15 percent a year. As the major community hospital on the north part of the island, NHCH offers a full range of traditional inpatient and outpatient services, including emergency care, intensive care, obstetrics/gynecology services, surgery for a variety of conditions, state-of-the-art imaging, home health care, skilled nursing care, dialysis treatment, rehabilitation services, telemedicine, and pain management. It has a women's center, a sleep laboratory, same-day surgery, and a family birthing unit. The hospital recently received the American Heart Association's (AHA) Get with the Guidelines–Coronary Artery Disease Initial Performance Achievement Award, which is given to hospitals where 85 percent of coronary patients are discharged following AHA-recommended treatments. NHCH also offers inpatients several types of CAM modalities, such as naturopathy, chiropractic care, acupuncture, and massage therapy.

In 2005, NHCH had 2,459 admissions, 551 deliveries, 11,313 emergency department visits, 31,581 outpatient visits, and 20,196 home care visits. Its annual operating budget was $26 million. Even though it is a busy community hospital, NHCH typically does not generate operating revenues sufficient to cover its costs. About 30 percent of hospital revenues come from Medicare, 12 percent from Medicaid, and 51 percent from private insurers, mostly from a single dominant insurer. NHCH attributes its financial problems to low payment rates for Medicaid in Hawaii and, especially, inadequate payments from the dominant private insurer. It has thus far been able to address its operating losses through philanthropy. For example, during its last fiscal year NHCH lost $1.4 million on operations but received a gift of land from the local Parker Ranch Foundation that more than offset the loss. (The hospital is one of four designated recipients for funds from the Parker Ranch Foundation.)

Philanthropy has played an important role in the short history of NHCH. The proposal to build NHCH was approved by the state legislature in 1991, with an estimated construction cost of $25 million. The state agreed to provide half the cost if the community raised the rest. As the planning process for constructing NHCH evolved, a consensus was achieved relatively quickly that it would not be "just another hospital." Instead, NHCH was designed "from the ground up" to be "patient centered" and congruent with Hawaiian cultural values and beliefs. Bakken, who had moved to Hawaii and was deeply involved in the development of the hospital, supported this vision and donated funds toward construction of the facility. Subsequently, he also provided funding for the purchase of cutting-edge medical equipment to help ensure that the hospital maintained a blend of "high-tech" and "high-touch" treatment capabilities. For example, his family foundation donated $3 million toward a $6.5 million, 4,000-square-foot imaging pavilion.[2]

The first CEO for the new hospital was recruited from an Arizona facility where he had helped to implement a "total healing environment" in which healing touch, guided imagery, and intentional breathing methods were provided for hospital patients.

Blended Medicine

The term "blended medicine" was coined by Earl Bakken, cofounder and director emeritus of Medtronic, a leading medical technology company and inventor of the first external, transistorized cardiac pacemaker in 1957. Bakken, now retired and living on the Big Island of Hawaii, was instrumental in helping build NHCH.

> I just think that people need to dream. I continually have dreams, just about every night, and believe that you have to carry out your dreams, literally. Some of them ... you can carry out quickly, and then some of them ... take more time. In 1978, I came up with the idea of "heart-brain medicine" and even organized a convention on the idea back then. But nothing happened. Now, almost 30 years later, we've got another convention coming up in Cleveland on heart-brain medicine, and this time ... I think it's going to catch on.
>
> Chronobiology is a perfect example. [As human beings] we have daily rhythms, weekly rhythms, 28-day rhythms, and annual rhythms. It is real science. And yet, people in this country are not using this knowledge. Why do they ignore it? By measuring someone's blood pressure for a week around the clock, you can predict from the blood pressure, the blood pressure amplitude, differences between systolic and diastolic pressures and the heart rate and rhythm, who is going to have a cardiovascular event. And when you know who is at risk for

an event, you have a much better opportunity for successful intervention.

"Ready ... Fire ... Aim" is one of the expressions that I live by. This is the approach I have used all my life. There are always decisions to be made. In my experience, it is better not to get caught up in the overanalysis of a problem. Many of the decisions at Medtronic were made quickly. The first pacemaker took only four weeks from concept to first use. The original design was not perfect, of course, but it worked!

PURSUING A PATIENT-ORIENTED STRATEGY

The stated vision of NHCH is "to treat the whole individual—mind, body, and spirit—through a team approach to patient-centered care, and ultimately to become the most healing hospital in the world." The facility built by the community was intended to be the foundation for achieving this vision.

Physical Environment

The design of NHCH as a supportive healing environment was a relatively unique undertaking in the early 1990's. The hospital makes extensive use of glass and skylights (even including windows in operating rooms) to bring natural light into the facility. Feng shui principles were employed in decisions relating to color, textures, and spatial relationships within the hospital. The fluorescent lighting was designed to avoid "flicker vision," power cables were buried more deeply than building codes require to reduce the effect of potentially harmful emissions, and a special water filtration system was installed for the hospital. Patient rooms are "oversized" to allow for family presence, and each room has a separate door to the outside as well as windows that open, to facilitate access to fresh air and sunshine and help reduce the "hospital smell." A separate room is available for families where they can rest, prepare meals, and play music. Hallways are relatively wide and are carpeted to reduce ambient noise levels. Spiritual icons representing the 14 main religions practiced by the hospital's patients are placed throughout the hospital. Outside the hospital is a healing garden, with flowers, trees, and water features, as well as a bamboo garden. A labyrinth garden is on the grounds for meditation. It features ceramic tiles depicting Hawaiian nature elements.[3] Taken together, these components of the physical environment are intended to put patients and their families at ease, facilitate patient healing, and support hospital staff in developing healing relationships with patients and each other.

Therapeutic Approach

Within this carefully designed physical environment, the goal of the hospital is to offer traditional and nontraditional treatment approaches in concert to achieve the best possible healing results for patients. Nontraditional approaches are available to hospitalized patients in two different ways. The first involves services provided as part of the hospital stay, at no cost to the patient. NHCH's Integrative Care Council, chaired by a physician and made up of 15 mid-level managers, has overall responsibility for supporting a healing environment in the hospital. Employees suggested the formation of the council to further enhance and promote the concept of blended medicine. The group self-selected and was approved by senior management. One individual, whose salary is funded outside the hospital's budget through philanthropy, holds the title of healing service leader and is a registered nurse and healing-touch practitioner. Her responsibility, she says, is "holding the vision of a healing environment in the hospital." She provides healing-touch therapy to about 40 percent of the hospital's patients, mostly in response to calls from nurses. For example, she may be called on to help relieve preoperative stress in patients or to assist in childbirths when labor is not progressing well. After the first treatment, she may be called back at the request of the patient. If time permits, she also goes "door to door" to offer her services. At one point, some physicians investigated the possibility of instituting an order process for her services, but they concluded that this was not necessary and that she could respond more rapidly without it. While her services now are provided largely without physician involvement, they are well received by most physicians.

The hospital also offers a limited array of complementary therapies (acupuncture, massage therapy, chiropractic care, aromatherapy) through providers who are credentialed to deliver the services in the hospital but are not hospital employees. This approach was favored by the hospital's medical staff and is consistent with the limited demand for these services. Recently, the hospital employed a massage therapist for a year, with costs underwritten by a gift. There did not appear to be enough potential revenue from this service to continue the massage therapist on staff after that year, however. Patients pay out of pocket for massage and acupuncture therapies, but private insurance typically reimburses for chiropractic care.

Challenges of Delivering Complementary Therapies at the Bedside

"There's always tension between the realities of hospital reimbursement, staff shortages, and the needs of the community with our vision for wanting to go beyond just routine hospital care. We're always seeking ways to bridge that gap. But in another way we are very fortunate. North Hawaii Community Hospital, with its beautiful natural setting and long, strong history and philosophy of being a healing environment, already exceeds the expectations of patients and care providers who have experienced other American hospitals."

Stan Berry, NHCH's CEO for the past five years maintains that managing patient expectations at his facility is not the difficult part. "They're not used to walking into a facility with the views that we have, the open spaces, the beautiful green mountains. They're not used to every room having a glass door or even the ICU having a large window, and all with garden views. They're not used to seeing the amount of artwork that we have in the hospital. Even the music, which is neither a popular or classical genre, but rather a unique, pleasant style, was developed especially for the hospital so as not to trigger any bad memories in patients. But when it comes to offering complementary therapies at the bedside, sometimes people have expectations we can't deliver on."

"Expectations can be both staff driven and patient driven. We attract a nursing team that really supports holistic care, and they'd like to see our patients have access to a broader range of services. But without physician support and sustainable reimbursement strategies, patients can't necessarily have a massage on request, acupuncture treatments to augment pain control, or a chiropractic adjustment from their own practitioner while they are in hospital."

Philanthropy has played a big part in the history of NHCH, which is not different from other hospitals that have been successful in creating healing environments.

Berry says, "We couldn't maintain this hospital without philanthropy because it allows us to bridge the gap between services provided and reimbursement. We have struggled for ten years to maximize our vision at NHCH, and even now, as I watch the rest of the world trying to catch up and see that everyone is interested in holistic care, I also see that nobody has yet figured out how to pay for it. Because our donor base is very generous, we're able to keep the buildings and grounds looking nice, and occasionally, there's money given to support holistic bedside care. But typically, donors want to build new facilities or buy equipment, not maintain programs." Berry observes that it is much harder to sell a concept like "healing environments" than it is to get a donor to buy a CT scanner or ICU monitor.

Spiritual Support

The hospital serves patients who practice a large number of different religions. According to the hospital's major benefactor, "We know we must honor each individual's basic human dignity and personal spiritual practices." The hospital's chapel is connected to the main building by a corridor and features natural light and an open view to the outdoors. Religious material for 14 different religions is available in the chapel. A "patient lavender" code is used in the hospital to alert staff to send a prayer or healing intention to a specific patient's room as needed. Members of the dietary staff are encouraged not to participate in food preparation if they are angry, because this would be contrary to "healing intention."

CHALLENGES TO THE STRATEGY

A general feeling permeates the hospital that its ability to invest in nontraditional services and healing touch is highly constrained by the operating deficits it experiences on a yearly basis. New initiatives and programs are not proposed because "everyone knows our situation." One consequence is that some new employees reportedly feel that the hospital "is not what it says it is" in regard to an innovative healing environment, nor is it reaching its full potential. Further, it is considered to be "in its infancy regarding integrating alternative services and creating whole-patient approaches," and its "reputation in the community exceeds its capacity to deliver regarding a healing environment."

Nevertheless, staff see hospital administrators as committed to the healing environment philosophy, even through changes in leadership. Leadership support is viewed in part as a response to the desires of hospital benefactors. But it is also seen as a response to the desires of the community, as evidenced by enthusiastic letters from patients and their families. The delivery of blended medicine in a unique healing environment remains an important factor in recruiting and retaining staff. However, it reportedly is less important for medical staff, who are challenged to treat "the whole patient" in an increasingly pressurized practice environment. Some physicians are said to be hesitant to try new approaches that might violate perceived standards of practice or invite malpractice litigation. Historically, no single physician has assumed the mantle of champion within the hospital for blended medicine and the mind/body/spirit approach to patient treatment espoused by the hospital.

While the investment in nontraditional services within NHCH has proceeded cautiously, several gains have been achieved in enhancing the high-tech side of blended medicine. The isolated location of NHCH and its small size pose significant challenges in this respect. However, the hospital has been able to leverage relationships established through its major benefactor, combined with the hospital's unique vision, to develop research projects and other initiatives. For example, in 2001 a researcher was recruited to NHCH to form the Department of Research. This researcher has made use of NHCH's state-of-the-art imaging equipment to study the effect of healing and prayer on the brain functions of recipients. In a second initiative, the University of Minnesota sends medical students to the hospital to be exposed to, and receive training in, a blended-medicine approach to care. Most recently, NHCH committed to establishing a heart-brain center. The center focuses attention and research on treating the heart and the brain as interconnected organs and caring for the whole body, rather than addressing only specific diseases or symptoms. The work of the center will be carried out jointly with the Cleveland Clinic, which will make its specialists available and work with NHCH to enhance its service capabilities.[4] This collaboration links NHCH with the Earl and Doris Bakken Heart-Brain Institute at the Cleveland Clinic, which was funded through a gift from NHCH's chief benefactor. A $12 million fund-raising campaign is now underway to build the heart-brain center at NHCH and upgrade related services.

KEYS TO SUCCESS

NHCH is now in its tenth year of implementing the vision of its founders that the hospital should provide a unique healing environment for its patients that blends the best of "high-tech" and "high-touch" treatment approaches in caring for the whole patient. While it continues to face significant challenges as it pursues this vision, it has also gained national attention for its efforts. Some of the keys to its success to this point follow.

Cultural Sensitivity and an Inspirational Vision

The hospital board, which is made up of community members, and the surrounding community support the hospital's vision. NHCH is a source of pride to the community and is seen as a desirable place to work. To a considerable extent, this community support derives from the hospital's efforts to respect local culture and religions in both its design and its day-to-day operations.

Beginning with a New Facility

The hospital started with a blank slate relative to physical plant. Consequently, in pursuing its vision it was not constrained by the limitations of an existing facility. It took advantage of this situation to design a hospital that was groundbreaking in its time. The new facility and its surroundings became a concrete representation of the hospital's vision for care, and, as intended, it continues to contribute to a supportive, healing environment for patients and for staff as well.

Philanthropy

Over time, the importance to NHCH of maintaining a continuing program of philanthropy has become abundantly clear. Given that the hospital is small and relatively isolated, philanthropy has been crucial to acquiring and updating cutting-edge treatment technology—the high-tech part of the hospital's vision—and collaborative relationships with external organizations. Ongoing philanthropy has also funded key aspects of the high-touch component of that vision. However, maintaining and increasing philanthropy for high-touch care is a continuing challenge.

ENDNOTES

1. North Hawaii Community Hospital (NHCH). 2006. "Welcome." [Online information; retrieved 3/21/07.] www.northhawaiicommunityhospital.org/index.html.

2. Enders, C. 2001. "Wise Medicine." *Insync* 21, p. 8.

3. Bakken, E. 2003. Presentation to the American College of Cardiology, October.

4. Stanton, K. 2006. "A Holistic Approach to Healing." *Hawaii Tribune Herald*, February 27, A1, A6.

CHAPTER 9

The Valley Hospital:
Reinvigorating Nursing at the Bedside

EXECUTIVE SUMMARY

The Valley Hospital (TVH) is a large community hospital located in Ridgewood, New Jersey. In 1998, under the leadership of a new chief nursing officer (CNO) and with the strong support of the hospital's CEO, it began to reconfigure the governance of nursing staff and redefine expectations around the nurse-patient relationship within the hospital. According to the CNO, "When I came to Valley, I felt the soul of nursing had atrophied and we needed to return to the core of nursing, which is the recognition of the need to care for the whole person—mind, body and spirit—including the nurse."[1]

Over the last eight years, she has launched a series of initiatives to address her concerns. These include a "shared governance" model for nursing, a training program in holistic practice for nurses (the Integrative Healing Arts Program), a holistic nursing council, a holistic practice nurse position, and the Center for the Advancement of Holistic Knowledge and Practice. While the transition was gradual over that period, it received a boost when TVH was awarded a grant from the Robert Wood Johnson Foundation in 2003 to evaluate a holistic nursing education initiative in the hospital. TVH has received national nursing awards for its efforts and now faces the challenge of expanding them within the hospital, and sustaining them financially.

BACKGROUND

TVH is an acute care, not-for-profit regional hospital that is part of the Valley Health System which, in addition to the hospital, includes Valley Home Care and Valley Health Medical Group (with approximately 20 physicians). TVH has 451 beds and, in 2005, had 50,677 admissions, 58,700 emergency department visits, and 3,205 deliveries. Measured by admissions, it is the second busiest hospital in New Jersey. TVH employs more than 3,500 people and has 1,450 volunteers. Approximately 1,100 physicians are on the medical staff, and 741 use the hospital as their preferred facility. The hospital employs about 1,300 nurses, 50 percent of whom are part time. Nurse turnover has declined from 15 percent annually eight years ago to 10 percent at present; one goal of TVH is to reduce this figure to 7 percent. Currently, TVH has a 2 percent vacancy rate for nurses.

The hospital offers a full range of services, including some of the latest surgical and imaging services, such as intensity-modulated radiation therapy for cancer care and video-assisted thoracic surgery for lung cancer. The Valley Columbia Heart Center is a joint effort of TVH, the New York–Presbyterian Healthcare System, and the Columbia University College of Physicians and Surgeons. Over the past two years, TVH has expanded its service lines, but these expansions typically have not occurred at the main campus. TVH faces capacity constraints, and growth potential at this campus, which is located in a residential area, is severely limited. As a consequence, in 2002 TVH opened a 128,000-square-foot facility in Paramus, New Jersey, that houses a variety of services, including a new cancer center. At present, TVH has six other facilities in addition to its primary location in Ridgewood.

TVH has recently received several national awards for its care and working environment. For example, it was designated a J.D. Power and Associates Distinguished Hospital for 2003, 2005, and 2006 for service excellence; named one of the 50 best places to work in New Jersey in 2005 and 2006; and achieved Magnet status for nursing excellence (the nursing profession's highest award) in 2003. In 2006 it was designated a winner of the 2006 Hospital of Choice Award by the American Alliance of Healthcare Providers, which recognizes "the nation's most consumer-friendly hospitals."[2]

The hospital's primary service area includes 32 towns and 440,000 people in Bergen County and neighboring counties. The area has 12 acute care hospitals and multiple outpatient surgery centers within a 15-mile radius of the hospital. TVH receives about 50 percent of its revenue from Medicare, 35 to 40 percent from private payers, and 1.4 percent from Medicaid. TVH characterizes its financial condition as "the best in the state" but anticipates that margins will shrink in the future due in part to competition from outpatient surgery centers. The medical staff is aging, so recruiting new physicians to the hospital to replace retiring physicians is becoming a priority.

PURSUING A PATIENT-ORIENTED STRATEGY

The mission statement for TVH places a strong emphasis on patient-centered care: "The Valley Hospital serves the community by healing and caring for patients, comforting their families and teaching good health." The pursuit of this mission took on a new focus with the arrival of a new CNO in 1998. Her goal was to strengthen nursing within the organization and reinvigorate the nursing staff by changing expectations regarding nursing care. She accomplished this goal through a variety of initiatives that built on each other and ultimately led TVH nurses "back to the future."

Repairing a Crack in the Foundation of Nursing

When Linda Cuoco, vice president for patient care and CNO, joined TVH, she found nurses who were withdrawn and, at the same time, concerned about nursing's future. Her challenge was to create a new model of nursing at TVH that would energize nurses and benefit patients.

I had been accustomed to very autonomous, spirited nursing professionals in my previous job roles, and with the reputation that Valley had in the community, I expected no less. To my surprise, I found a very much disheartened corps of nurses. What I learned over the first 30 days in my role was that, indeed, their heart and spirit for their profession was "atrophied." In fact, I shared with my CEO that I felt there was a "giant crack in the foundation of nursing" and the level of care and clinical outcomes [were] beginning to show the decline. We were at the 46th percentile in patient satisfaction, and the RN turnover rate was close to 15 percent. All were signs of a disheartened team. Over the next 90 days, I spent time with the staff and leadership trying to understand and learn what they were all about. This is what I learned. For the previous several years, the organization had embraced (or at least senior management) the movement of redesign. The [redesign] process [resulted in] changed roles so that patients had as few people encounters as possible during their hospitalization. Nursing roles were changed [due to the redesign] to oversee all support care, including housekeeping, blood draws, transportation, and "other duties" as needed.

Their titles were [also] changed [as part of the redesign process] from RNs to clinical associates, like every other clinical professional in the organization. In fact, it appeared that only nurses had their functional roles significantly changed compared to others in the organization. Their roles [had become] confusing, both to them and to their patients, and this lead to confusion, frustration, and a decrease in pride.

My work was to establish a clear direction to rebuild the pride and professionalism of nursing. Through their willingness and openness to share, we created lists of what was working well and what was not working well. This was the foundation for my action plan. We created, together, the shared governance foundation in which all of nursing could have a voice, take charge of their profession, and create their future. This was only the beginning. I knew their heart was in need of a reawakening of spirit and pride for their profession. They needed and wanted to feel like they were once again doing real "hands on" nursing, being with their patients, teaching, comforting, and healing. I wanted to cocreate a nursing culture that would produce and sustain the type of nurse-healer that I would want to take care of me and my family in the future. Together with consultants from the Birchtree Center, we created the Integrative Healing Arts Program, which set the principles and foundation for our holistic practice today.

Adoption of a Shared Governance Model

Beginning in 1998, TVH increased the nurses' level of involvement in decision making related to nursing practice matters such as autonomy, organizational support, and relationships with medical staff. In 2000, this approach was formalized by enacting a shared governance model. The stated goal of the model is "to develop our professional staff so that they, in collaboration with management, share all responsibilities for the evolution of patient care practices within a holistic framework."[3] The model reinforces the important role of nurses within the organization. The change in composition of key governing "councils" indicates the high degree of adoption of the model. For example, "In 1998, the Nurse Practice Education Council comprised all management and advanced practice nurses. Today, the Nurse Practice Council is 90 percent frontline staff and the Performance Improvement Council is 95 percent frontline staff."[4]

Service Excellence Initiative

The service excellence initiative created a leadership training program within the hospital. Its goal was to facilitate leadership development and a common, supportive leadership culture throughout all parts of the organization.

Integrative Healing Arts Program

TVH established its Integrative Healing Arts Program in 2001. The purpose of the program was to train nursing staff, on a voluntary basis, in the skills they need to "return" to a mind/body/spirit approach to nursing practice. These include techniques to help patients manage pain, relax, and manage anxiety.[5] The cost is $1,500 to $2,000 per student, with approximately 20 students per class. The hope is that, over time, all of the nurses at TVH will receive training in holistic practices, but it is not expected that all will complete the entire 18-month program. The techniques nurses learn in this training program are intended to become an integral part of patient care. Nurses do not require a physician order to apply these techniques at the bedside, nor are their efforts treated as billable services.

Robert Wood Johnson Foundation Grant

In 2003, TVH receive a two-year grant from the Robert Wood Johnson Foundation (RWJF) to test whether a nursing education and practice model, based on promoting a "caring culture" and nursing autonomy, could increase nurse job satisfaction and improve recruitment and retention. Two units within the hospital were selected as pilot sites, and nursing staff were invited to participate in the Integrative Healing Arts Program. Staff members were given four days of release time for the program and were not available on their units during this time. Fifty percent of the nursing staff in each unit had completed the program by March 2005. Compared with those of control units, nurse turnover rates were lower and patient satisfaction higher in the pilot units, but the number of individuals involved was small, and differences were not statistically significant. Nevertheless, management was particularly interested in the reduction in nurse turnover in the pilot units, because of its potential implications for reducing the costs of recruiting and training new nurses.[6]

Holistic Practice Council

The Holistic Practice Council was added to the hospital's shared governance structure in March 2004. As one of its responsibilities, the council oversees the integration of holistic nursing practices across TVH. All policies and procedures relating to these practices are reviewed by the council, which then makes recommendations to the Nurse Practice Education Council and, ultimately, the Patient Care Services Leadership Council. The formation of the Holistic Practice Council in effect institutionalizes the hospital's commitment to a holistic approach to nursing care.

Holistic Practitioner Position

In June 2004, TVH hired its first holistic practitioner, a newly created position. This person works in conjunction with nurses in the hospital units to incorporate various principles and techniques into patient care, including guided imagery, breath work, and therapeutic touch techniques. Besides providing these services directly to patients, the practitioner serves as a bridge to assist nurses in carrying their healing arts training into practice. Twelve TVH nurses have achieved national certification as holistic nurses through the American Holistic Nurses Credentialing Corporation and now provide care to patients on the unit where they work. At any one time, the holistic practitioner herself may be providing services to 15 to 20 hospitalized patients.

At the TVH Leadership Institute in October 2004, the holistic practitioner, joined by a harpist, demonstrated the use of guided imagery therapy for stress reduction. The session was so well received that a guided imagery CD was created based on it. In 2005, the hospital created a second holistic practitioner position. The holistic practitioner sets aside about two hours on Fridays to activities designed to reduce stress in nurses, so that they can experience how these same techniques can be used in the treatment of their patients.

Center for the Advancement of Holistic Knowledge and Practice

The hospital created its Center for the Advancement of Holistic Knowledge and Practice in May 2005. The mission of the center is "Advocating for the advancement of holistic knowledge and practice by serving as mentors to health care professionals facilitating the growth of holistic education and evidence-based practice and research." The center provides ongoing education and training to TVH staff in patient care practices such as the use of aromatherapy, therapeutic touch, and meditation. These classes are taught primarily by staff members who have completed the Integrative Healing Arts Program. The center manages the Healing Arts Program and it contracts with external vendors for training in various techniques where necessary, coordinating its efforts with the hospital's Center for Complementary Therapy and TVH's education departments.

In addition to these initiatives, which are directed at implementing what TVH calls a "holistic approach" to nursing practice, the hospital has several other ongoing efforts to support patients, families, and nurses. One of these efforts, the Harp Music Therapy Program, is highly visible within the hospital. Under this program, "a harpist plays at or near the bedside of patients whom the staff identify as being good candidates for this kind of relaxation therapy."[7] The harp music can have a tension-relieving impact on nursing staff as well as patients. A second initiative, the Center for Complementary Therapy, primarily serves the surrounding community and patients after they are discharged from the hospital. The center offers classes in areas such as stress management, yoga, and guided imagery. Individuals can also visit the center to receive acupuncture therapy, counseling in smoking cessation, and therapeutic massage. Unlike the services provided by nurses at the bedside for hospitalized patients, individuals pay separately for the center's services, which are delivered on an outpatient basis.

CHALLENGES TO THE STRATEGY

The holistic nursing practice effort is supported indirectly at TVH by a "rewards for results" program aimed at improving patient satisfaction scores. If quarterly patient satisfaction targets are met and hospital financial targets are reached, each hospital employee receives a $100 bonus (for a total of about $300,000 across the organization per quarter). Financing the holistic nursing practices initiatives has not been a major issue to this point. The holistic nurse practitioner is included in the hospital's budget, along with the cost of training nurses in holistic care. (Training costs are included in each unit's education budget.) The evidence from the RWJF grant that nurse turnover may be reduced under this approach is seen by hospital leaders as an indicator that financial benefits from the approach probably exceed costs.

The Impact of Holistic Nursing at TVH:
A Financial Perspective

"A hospital is nothing without an adequate number of experienced, well-educated, highly motivated registered nurses. There is no job category in a hospital that contributes more to patient outcomes and satisfaction, the hospital's reputation within the local community, and ultimately, its overall success than the registered nurses."

With those statements as a backdrop, Richard Keenan, the chief financial officer of TVH explains why he views the holistic nursing initiative at TVH as "an unqualified success."

This program started in 2001 at an initial cost of $25,000. Then, through a Robert Wood Johnson Foundation grant, the research began with the two pilot units in 2003.

The overall objectives of the holistic nursing program were to

- improve patient outcomes and satisfaction,
- increase the job satisfaction of the staff registered nurses,
- reduce staff RN turnover,
- enhance the hospital's ability to recruit both new graduates and experienced nurses, [and]
- reduce the use of temporary staff (agency nurses).

The initiative was called the Integrative Healing Arts Program and was introduced on two medical/surgical units. The results were dramatic and quickly evident:

- A substantial reduction in RN turnover, which was as high as 13.5 percent in 2000. It dropped to 9.5 percent in 2005. The two pilot units averaged only 7 percent for the year 2005, and for the study period (24 months), each had zero turnover. With the cost of losing and replacing one full-time RN estimated at $50,000, the reduction in turnover alone more than offset the cost of implementation.

- The RN vacancy rate went from 6.5 percent in 2002 to virtually zero in 2005.
- Agency nurse usage, which averaged $3 million to $5 million in recent years, fell to less than $150,000 in 2005. The agency staff who were used in 2005 were nursing assistants used as "sitters" to maintain a restraint-free environment.
- Employee satisfaction increased from the 60th percentile in 2000 to the 85th percentile in 2003 to the 90th percentile in 2006.
- Patient satisfaction has increased from the 83rd percentile in 2000 to the 96th percentile in 2006.
- All patient outcome measures, such as falls, medication errors, and infection rates, are setting new record lows.

Admittedly, holistic nursing was carried out along with other activities, but its contribution to achieving the dramatic improvement in the above-noted metrics is unquestionable. Some other initiatives were the following:

- Shared governance, which gave nurses a voice and the ability to better influence their daily work environment
- Bridges to Belonging, a retention strategy directed toward new employees.

Although the holistic nursing initiative was carried out with other activities, no one who observed its impact doubts its contribution to the overall results and that the program added value far above the minimal cost of implementation.

Going forward, the Center for Holistic Knowledge and Practice hopes to generate revenue to support its work by charging fees for courses provided to nurses and others from outside the Valley Health System who want to learn holistic practice techniques.

Generally, the development of a holistic approach to nursing has been well received by TVH nurses, but in the beginning a significant number of nurses thought aspects of the approach were "silly." For instance, as part of the RWJF grant, nurses in the pilot units were asked to practice the "setting of intention" at the start of their shifts. This is described as a "technique of using one's thoughts to visualize a positive outcome and setting one's intention to align thought and action."[8] During this process, nurses typically held hands and, for example, stated their intention to support one another in the care of a particularly complex patient. Some nurses resisted participating in the setting of intention at the start of their shifts, believing it to be "too much like praying." Over time, much of this concern dissipated and setting of intention is now carried out, in various forms, at the beginning of many meetings involving nursing staff.

A more fundamental problem for nurses arises when staffing shortages occur, which normally has not been a significant issue at TVH. When they do occur, however, time constraints can result in nurses feeling as though they do not have enough time to spend with patients to provide healing touch or guided-imagery therapies. Also, when nurses trained in the holistic approach move to other units or positions within the hospital, such change can slow the momentum for adopting holistic practices in the units they leave.

Physicians at TVH are reported to be largely indifferent to efforts to implement holistic nursing practices. Some nursing managers believe this is because the changes have occurred gradually over time. Physicians have had little direct involvement, as they do not need to order these practices for their patients. This could change if, in the future, TVH begins to incorporate CAM practices into inpatient care. Occasionally, individual physicians have become vocal supporters of holistic nursing practices, because they have seen exceptional results when techniques such as healing touch have been used with their patients.

KEYS TO SUCCESS

TVH has attempted, over an eight-year period, to change the focus of nursing with the goal of creating a stronger healing relationship between nurses and patients at the bedside. This effort has been largely successful to this point, and TVH is now attempting to expand holistic nursing to all units and to develop an approach that will make CAM more easily accessible for hospitalized patients who wish these services. There appear to be four keys to TVH's success.

Vision and Support of Hospital Leadership

A strong consensus exists within the hospital that the most important factor in TVH's success has been the vision and support of hospital leadership. The hospital's CNO, with strong backing from the CEO, is credited with creating and executing a plan to change nursing practice in the hospital while developing support for that plan among the hospital's nurses.

Gradual Implementation

Nursing practice changes occurred gradually over the eight-year period. This allowed nurses to grow in their abilities to participate in a shared governance model and to develop a sense of ownership of the changes. It also minimized the potential for opposition on the part of TVH's physicians and provided opportunities for physician leaders to observe the benefits of the changes for their patients.

Controlling Costs

None of the steps taken to change nursing practice have required significant new funding. Because of their gradual implementation, they have not raised major concerns in the annual budget process. Now, attention is being focused on the potential cost savings from these practices in the form of increased nurse retention rates.

External Grant Support

The grant from RWJF did not alter the direction of the hospital with respect to its efforts to change nursing practice. However, it did accelerate the process and focus attention on nursing practices within the hospital. The grant also encouraged the measurement and tracking of outcomes. Most outcomes were positive, which underscored the validity of the approach.

ENDNOTES

1. Assi, M. J., and M. Shanahan. 2005. "Holistic Care & Nursing Science: Retaining Magnet Excellence" *Excellence in Nursing Knowledge*. January. [Online publication; retrieved 5/1/07]. www.nursingknowledge.org

2. The Valley Hospital (TVH). 2007. "About The Valley Hospital." [Online information; retrieved 3/21/07.] www.valleyhealth.com.

3. TVH. 2005. "Patient Care Services: Shared Management." Internal document.

4. TVH (2005).

5. Kinsley, M. 2006. "The Magic of Touch." *Nursing Spectrum*, New York/New Jersey Metro Edition, January 16, pp. 10–11.

6. Assi, M. J. 2006. "Final Narrative Report." The Valley Hospital internal document, January 31.

7. Kinsley (2006).

8. ENK (2005).

CHAPTER 10

Putting the Components of a Reinvented Patient Experience in Place

This chapter contains a portion of the edited transcript of a day-long roundtable discussion involving representatives from seven of the eight hospitals described in Chapters 2 through 9. The roundtable provided an opportunity for these innovators to exchange ideas and information concerning their experiences implementing patient-focused strategies in their organizations. This chapter is structured around discussion of four areas of patient-focused innovation that were identified through a cross-organizational analysis of the eight study hospitals: physical environment, nursing practices, complementary therapies, and spiritual support.

In preparation for the roundtable, specific individuals were asked to share experiences in each area, and others were invited to comment or react. The discussion was facilitated by Michael Finch, Ph.D., one of the project researchers. The following were participants in the discussion:

Stan Berry, president and CEO, North Hawaii Community Hospital

Linda Cuoco, vice president, Patient Care Services, and CNO,
The Valley Hospital

Michael Finch, senior fellow and consultant, Optimal Healing
Environments, Samueli Institute

Grace Henley, assistant administrator, Human Resources,
Highline Medical Center

Lori Knutson, director, Institute for Health and Healing,
Abbot Northwestern Hospital

Kathy Mitchell, CNO, Adventist Bolingbrook Medical Center

Nancy Moore, vice president, Healing Health Services, and
CNO, St. Charles Medical Center

Vicki VanMeetren, president, St. Rose Dominican
Hospitals–San Martín Campus

MR. FINCH: We've asked Nancy to start off by briefly telling us about St. Charles in terms of transforming care at the bedside.

MS. MOORE: St. Charles operates under a healing healthcare philosophy. The ethic of the philosophy is healing ourselves, our relationships, our community. So it starts with us, you know, the people that work there. One of the things we say is that we're a human service. We're people caring for people. We don't make hotdogs or automobiles. And so, to the extent that the hospital staff themselves are whole and well and healed, they can be present in a healing way for other people. When our caregivers are healthy, and they're working in a healthy relationship with each other, then patients receive good care.

So I would say the essence of what we're doing in transforming care at the bedside is about relationships and relationship-centered care. People don't necessarily learn good communication skills in their family of origin. And some may have learned them, but when they go to school it gets trained out of them. Some of our physicians have told us that. So we offer a personal growth and development workshop that's two-and-a-half days that is part of orientation. The skills that come out of that workshop involve greater self-awareness and healthy communication. I would say that's a major part of transforming care at the bedside.

We also have designed our facility around care at the bedside. In our newest construction, there is one nursing station for every four rooms, and it's right outside the patients' doors so that the caregivers are decentralized to the patients' rooms. They're at the bedside versus out in the nurses' station. All the supplies are there, the medications are there, and the equipment is there. There is a place to store IV poles and pumps and things in the room to try to reduce all the steps and all the activities that physically take the caregiver away from the patient.

The other aspect is providing therapeutic interventions that enhance healing. We have what we call Healing Health Care resources; they're methods to reduce anxiety and pain and enhance relaxation. We created core competencies in these methods that are required by every caregiver, and examples include intentional breathing, guided imagery, and relaxation methods. In addition a number of nurses are trained in therapeutic touch. They also receive education on when to refer to physical therapy, social service, or spiritual care. We also have a prayer procedure that guides everybody in how to offer prayer in a way that's respectful to people's belief systems if that's what they want.

These kinds of therapies really are available any time to the patient. We believe that enhances their healing response, because when they're relaxed, their natural healing responses work. When they're stressed and scared, they shut down and healing is impaired. We found out we really needed to have Healing Health Care resource mentors on each unit to keep those skills alive and available for people. It didn't work to have that centralized. It really needed to be on the units. It's additional duties for someone, most often a nurse, who has special training. These Healing Health Care resource mentors make sure all their team members are trained in those skills and keep the referral list for therapeutic touch current.

We have Internet access in the patient's room for families, and computers and family resource centers where patients and families can go on the Internet or they can print out education in lay terms related to their medication or their illness.

Putting pharmacists on the units has been important as well. We have a decentralized pharmacy. Pharmacists are making rounds with physicians and nurses, and they are responding to drug interactions and addressing those specialized meds that really benefit from their expertise in doing the patient education.

We also have a health and learning center where people can access our prevention and wellness services. The center offers a number of programs, from a six-week managing chronic symptoms program based on Stanford University's psychoeducational model to support groups and medication classes. When a person needs to be admitted to the hospital, nurses are expected to have a therapeutic relationship throughout the patient's stay, and other disciplines are involved as needed. When patients are discharged they are referred to the programs in the health and learning center or other community resources as appropriate.

With respect to nursing, we have a minimum service standard called the caring model. It is based on creating a discipline where nurses sit down with patients for five minutes, introduce themselves, describe their role in their care, ask patients how they like to be addressed and what their most important needs are, what's most important to them, and what they would like to have accomplished today and during their stay. And then the nurses make sure that it gets documented and addressed. There are grease boards in the room where they write the nurse's name as well as the patient's needs and goals down so everybody knows. And they use appropriate touch. We also expect that they will use the mission and values in planning patients' care. It's so basic but it wasn't happening consistently, and it continues to require ongoing monitoring and reinforcement.

This is all based on our Healing Health Care philosophy. We also reinforce that all departments support patient- and family-focused care. Other departments, such as finance and facilities services, may not physically touch the patient as nurses do, but what they do makes a difference in patients' care. We expect department managers to translate for their department's caregivers how their work contributes to patient care.

MS. CUOCO: I joined The Valley Hospital in 1998 at a time that the hospital was a premier hospital in northern New Jersey. When you're a brand new CNO and they tell you how wonderful the hospital is, and they have such a great reputation, you believe it. Well, I found that nursing, which is the founding service of any hospital, was broken.

The hospital had been through years of redesign, and the spirit of nursing was gone. In my first report to the board, after 45 days, I told them that they had a broken engine. And they looked at me and said, "No, we're a premier hospital." But you could see it in outcomes. The clinical outcomes were not as good as they should be. Patient satisfaction at that time was in the 46th percentile. Even though the hospital had a wonderful image, it was still broken.

I decided that one of the first things you have to do is rebuild that foundation, and so that's how holistic practice came about. In 2000, we launched the first healing arts program. We'd always done workshops, but never had launched them with the intent of changing the practice of nursing, and that's what we've been able to do at Valley.

One of the things we were able to do early on is to get a Robert Wood Johnson Foundation grant, which actually catapulted us to where we are today. We were able to do two primary nursing units, taking them through an 18-month course. The course teaches everything from self-care, which is probably the most important piece, all the way to modalities like aromatherapy, music therapy, and body work therapy.

As a CNO, you have to speak in a language that your board understands and your CEO understands. I kept our efforts quiet for quite some time. Now we have a very robust system for holistic practice. I have 12 nationally certified advanced practice nurses, and half of them are nurse practitioners, but they're also nationally certified in holistic practice.

Last year, we launched the Center for Advancement of Holistic Knowledge and Practice, which is an education center. Out of about 1,500 registered nurses, we only have about 200 who have gone through the program in its entirety. We decided this year to launch it in small segments. We're doing eight-hour courses for all of the registered nurses and four-hour courses for all the support staff. Through that process, we hope to make sure over time that every nurse in the organization gets through orientation, and every nurse who has been there will have this kind of training under his or her belt.

With respect to results, we went from the 46th percentile in 2000 all the way to the 94th percentile of Press Ganey, which is our patient satisfaction service. And this year we're hovering around the 96th percentile. With respect to employee satisfaction, we went from the 60th percentile of Press Ganey to the 94th percentile. My nurse vacancy rate in 2000 was horrendous, and now we've dropped down to .05, and we're in a very highly competitive area. I not only have the New York hospitals 40 minutes away from me, but I also have very outstanding institutes just a stone's throw away.

I'll just give you a normal day's picture. The morning starts with setting of intentions, a one- or two-minute gathering of the troops to say this is going to be a very busy day, we need to sit together, we need to make sure everybody goes on breaks. And someone—each of the staff members has that opportunity—but someone brings something inspirational. We keep it away from being religious. We're a nondenominational organization, but we try to keep it spiritual and uplifting. And sometimes that's kind of hard because it's really easy to go into the religious side. It seems very comfortable for everyone around the table to do that.

After the morning starts, usually at about 11:30 in the morning, a chime goes through the organization. When you hear that chime you take a minute, take a deep breath, wherever you are, just stop. We launched that last year. We're not quite getting everybody to stop, but we're working on it. We believe that everyone should stop for a moment and think about what they're doing and how to be a better team, how to approach their patients in a kinder fashion. We also started a healing time for our patients. It happens at 8 o'clock in the evening when we turn our lights low in all of the inpatient areas, and people are asked to be very quiet for one hour. Either light music is played or, depending on what the unit is, bedside care is delivered. It's the old-fashioned PM care that we all grew up with as nurses. In essence, it's hands on. It's doing some kind of body work. Aromatherapy goes on during that quiet hour.

There are 200 of us in the organization who have been taught the "M" technique, which is a body-work therapy that is done in three rhythmic strokes. It's usually done with jojoba oil and lavender if the patient would like that. If not, it's just done with warm lotion. We work on the hands and feet primarily. We also do music therapy.

We have a bedside harp program that was launched three years ago. It's a beautiful melody, a beautiful tone, and it's very healing. We have harp students who go through the organization at all times, and then of course we have master harpists who are the trainers of the program, and you'll just see them strolling around the organization.

We also have a music listening program. Our music therapist has developed music listening programs on all of the units to help nurses understand how to use music therapeutically, when is the right time and place, and how you do that. And we've incorporated the Care Channel. We encourage patients to use the Care Channel when they first come into their room, when they're about ready to go off for a test of some sort, or anytime when there is a sense that anxiety is beginning to be aroused.

We have a 40-hour intensive training course that we're calling our Nurse Liaison Program. It's bedside nurses, who receive this intensive training over a year. They receive 40 hours of classroom training that's both lecture based and experiential, and they learn some skills. And then, for the following year, they are mentored by our nurse clinicians at the bedside to learn how to put their training into practice. The mentorship program is the newest part of what we're doing, and I think it's probably been the most significant part of truly integrating holistic care at the bedside.

We were working with staff nurses on massage because it's not so foreign to most of the nurses; the use of guided imagery and understanding this whole psychoneural immunology component; and then several different relaxation techniques. Those are the primary tools that we use. But we talk about understanding the philosophy, about what it means to do these therapies, that they're not just tasks, and that there's meaning and purpose in what you do in connection with the patient. That is fundamental to all the training that we provide for them.

MR. BERRY: I'd like to ask a question. Did you have unions at either place that you had to deal with?

MS. CUOCO: No, but I have unions all around me. In fact, the most interesting part is that unions have really identified New Jersey as a pivotal place. The holistic practice is one of those things that has actually kept unions at bay because this really hits the heart of nursing.

MR. BERRY: We're nonunion but I see around me the antagonism that exists. The unions want to sell their product as if they're the big defender of nursing, and they sort of want to fossilize things that don't make a lot of sense.

MS. KNUTSON: We are from a union hospital. We engaged the union at the very beginning to have them buy in on it and have them participate in it, and now they're our big champions. In fact, they want to create language around negotiations about holistic nursing.

MS. MOORE: In Oregon, the Oregon Nurses' Association has a very strong labor arm, so most of the hospitals in Oregon are unionized. Our RNs are in the Oregon Nurses' Association Union. I don't think it's necessarily an obstacle. It's another entity that you have a relationship with.

MR. BERRY: How do your nursing ratios look? California has 1 to 5 for med-surg, for instance, 1 to 2 in ICU. Are you in that ballpark?

MS. CUOCO: We're actually not as good as that. We sit about 1 to 6 on a med-surg unit and 1 to 4, 1 to 5 on interventional units. Over the years I've added about 25 percent more bedside nurses. One of the biggest push-backs that I got from the staff nurses was, "When are we going to have enough time, Linda, to do this one more thing?" And interesting enough, when they want to do something, the time is found, and you actually see a better patient outcome.

One of the things we implemented was hourly rounding. When asked to see patients on an hourly basis, nurses will say they don't have enough time. But we actually have given them time back. Each time they say they don't have enough staff, you work with them and they find out that if you change some things, you do have time. I would certainly like to add more staff. We just don't have the budget to do that.

MR. BERRY: Do you have nursing aides and ward clerks that provide support, transporters, and so forth?

MS. CUOCO: We sure do. We have transport. For a 25-bed unit, we'll have three techs, which are equivalent to nurse's aides on the West Coast. Those techs draw blood and do EKGs, and they'll do supportive care baths and other care. But the majority of the work still falls on the nurse.

I just wanted to talk about our physicians. Probably my biggest advocates are a critical care intensivist and the president of the medical staff. Again, I never asked permission. I always put into practice things that are well within the scope of nursing, and I don't have to ask permission. If you just let it permeate, it gets through much faster. What really turned around that intensivist was that several years ago he had a patient who he could not stabilize. One of the things I forgot to tell you is I also have two physicians, full-time physicians, that are advance practice nurses who are nationally certified in holistic practice and also instructors for aromatherapy, body work therapy, and the end technique. Their total job is to go throughout the organization for referrals to do some real hands-on with the patients. And luckily enough, they happened to be in critical care one day when the intensivist was up there just trying to stabilize this patient, and having great difficulty.

So the nurse went to the bedside, pulled the curtains and, as the physicians talked about the next round of events for this patient, they noticed on the external monitor that the vital signs had begun to stabilize. They couldn't understand why the patient's heart rate was returning to normal. So, long story short, they said, "well, what's going on?" So the intensivist tested, the next time, and the next time, and kept testing. And now, as soon as he has a patient he's not able to manage, he calls the nurse in early.

MS. MOORE: Probably about 40 percent of our physicians have been through our people-centered team training. Sometimes it's individualized for them. At one of our larger, multispecialty clinics we did a special class that was just one day instead of the usual two-and-a-half days. One of the physicians in that large multispecialty clinic was very much against the holistic nursing approach—he was the medical director for the Emergency Services Department. During that seminar he awakened to why he went into medicine and became one of our biggest champions for mind/body/spirit care. We've had about five or six of those situations, and that has spread out to other physicians.

MR. FINCH: Can you talk a little bit about the challenges that implementing electronic medical records poses or creates for you in terms of maintaining this approach to nursing?

MS. MOORE: We implemented our electronic medical record and computerized physician order entry in October of 2004. It was a huge, huge transformative event. We knew it would be big, but it was so much bigger than we anticipated because it included physician order entry. Everybody had to change their mental structure of thinking. And it did create a barrier between the caregiver and the patient. It may have been because of our planning. Yet I don't know if it would have helped had we implemented it differently. We want the nurses to take the computer into the room with them and treat it as a part of the experience. Where we have nurses doing that, and they show the patient their vital signs, a graph of their pulse, a temperature coming down, it's a part of the healing experience.

But we haven't got the nurses to where they're comfortable. Because of their insecurity with the system, they have been hesitant to include it as part of the care experience. It takes more time, so nurses feel like they have less time for holding a patient's hand, for sitting down and talking with patients, than they had before. I'm doing a work study to analyze how the nurses are now spending their time. We will use this information to make improvements that allow more time for direct patient care.

MS. VANMEETREN: In our system, which we are implementing, we don't take it to the bedside. We've built a visual aid right outside the room, and our physicians sit there. They know the medical record's there so they don't have to go searching for it. The interesting thing is that our patients, if they forget a question for the doctor, will just come out because they see him there. They'll say, "Excuse me, Dr. Jones, but there was one more question we forgot."

Physicians also use it as an educational tool. I see physicians pointing on the screen and families gathered around. And the physicians actually feel comfortable away from the desk, sitting right there outside the room. But in the patient room it was perceived by the caregivers as invasion of privacy if the family's talking.

MS. MITCHELL: I think we have to give nurses options and tools to work with on the patient care unit, and let them decide what they feel good using, whether they want to sit in that space that you've designed, or whether they want to bring the computer into the room to collect information and bring it out. I think it's different from individual to individual, and we are probably going to have to accept that. We learned that you can't have a tool in the patient room for the patient to use for entertainment and to access the Web, and for the caregiver to use as well. Patients need their device and the staff needs their devices—and never the two shall mix. I'm pretty sure about that.

MS. CUOCO: We've been struggling with whether the computer should be at the bedside or in the stations or in cubicles or alcoves. Every nurse is a little bit different. Some feel like it's an invasion of their ability to do their work well if they have to be told to be at the bedside. Hopefully, we'll go to notebooks or handhelds eventually. When you're doing a full assessment, sometimes it takes quite a lengthy amount of time, and so nurses would rather be sitting someplace and doing that.

One of the things we're looking at in designing a new tower is centralized nursing stations. When I came into the organization, and it was using decentralized pods, I found that many times people didn't talk to each other, and so the community of nursing was more fragmented than need be. I have a combination of pods and a central station. I find the community and the camaraderie between physicians and nurses are much stronger when they meet in the primary station. I encourage them to have social discussions because this breaks down the walls between doctors and nurses. So I've been supporting both having a central station for that socialization and then decentralized work areas. It's worked out well.

MR. BERRY: Do you have any cultural push-backs by patients who don't want to be touched or have their feet rubbed?

MS. CUOCO: Absolutely.

MR. BERRY: So you just make sure they understand those things?

MS. CUOCO: Nurses say to the patient that they can help the patient relax. "If you'd like, we can put oil on your feet and rub them." A few people say they don't want their feet touched. Then, we just put a little music on and put a little aromatherapy at the bedside. We can accomplish quite a bit with that, too.

MR. FINCH: With respect to nursing practice at the bedside, are these things transportable to other hospitals?

MS. CUOCO: That was the premise of the Robert Wood Johnson grant. It had to be transportable. And so we studied how much money it would cost and all of that. And I will tell you it's a combination of both good people and a good program.

MS. VANMEETREN: I think those people who don't fit, leave.

MS. MOORE: Yes, I agree.

MS. VANMEETREN: And so the culture attracts the kind of people who feel very comfortable in that setting.

When we have our orientation, we have a day of "values in action," it's called. And at the end of that day, there is role playing about how you get along with people. It concludes with a sister pretty much saying that if this feels odd to you, then probably you don't belong here. It doesn't mean that we're saying go away; it just means don't be embarrassed if this is odd. Everyone is basically just about taking care of the patient. Every patient is someone that you give courtesy and care to. We expect you to walk someone to their destination, not to say, "Go down the hall, turn left." If that seems odd, then maybe you don't belong here.

MR. FINCH: Let's move on to our next topic, which is making complementary therapies available to patients.

MS. KNUTSON: Currently, we have an inpatient program related to health and healing. We have six nurse clinicians who are full time. Fifty percent of their position is to do education of staff nurses and ancillary departments, and the other 50 percent of their position is direct patient care. So they get referrals, and they go out and see patients. They are all holistic nurses, and all come with a specialty background. So, for instance, the nurse who is in cardiovascular care is a 25-year veteran intensive care nurse. The nurse that I have in women's care is a clinical nurse specialist in women's care, and she's a holistic nurse. They're all certified in a multitude of different kinds of complementary therapies. So they come with a tool bag. Plus, they have the language to speak and sort of translate these therapies into conventional medicine. They are partnered with a full-time acupuncturist and a full-time massage therapist.

Our hospital has nine centers of excellence, and we are fully operational in six of the nine. I have groups in med-surg, oncology, cardiovascular care, women's care, neurology, orthopedics, and rehabilitation. We have a music therapist on staff, and we have a multitude of practitioners that help to fill in on a part-time basis according to referrals.

We started out with really focusing on what nurses could provide at the bedside, because we knew that was the most straightforward way for us to really get it implemented. For it to be sustainable, nurses had to be engaged in the process of complementary therapies.

From there, I'll jump to the present. We now have physicians from all those centers of excellence who are champions. They are the medical directors of the centers of excellence, and they are our advisory team to the Institute for Health and Healing. Having that physician partnership was crucial for us to be totally in the fabric of the hospital environment. We have partnerships with them right now, and it's working incredibly well.

We also have an outpatient center, where we do referrals to the outpatient environment, and a new fitness center that we're just getting started. Fundamentally, for us it's not about complementary therapies; it's about nutrition, it's about exercise, and it's about mind and body therapies. More deeply than that, it is how the mind and the body interface in the biochemistry of what's going on. So those are the fundamental pieces. We offer whatever therapy seems to be the right therapy at that time to connect with the patient. In some cases, all that is needed is communication. It's sitting with the patient, holding the patient's hand or not holding the hand, depending on what the patient's culture is.

I have to say we've learned a lot from the cultures that we've served. We've had patients from many cultures come back and give us in-services, and it has been phenomenal for us to have that experience.

When we started out, we followed the vision and the mission of Allina Health Systems and the vision and the mission of Abbott Northwestern Hospital. How do we speak to that in the work we want to bring forward? How do we look at the financials around what the organization wants to do, and how can we impact that? I'll give you one example of how we worked with a physician who really was not supportive. He had problems with patients not being able to sit through certain tests. He was not looking too good in his practice because patients' lengths of stay were increasing. Most of this was due to patient anxiety relating to the tests. So we offered to have somebody available for every treatment, so that we could help in reducing anxiety. The patient then followed through with the treatment. In a short period of time, that physician became a champion, because he saw that patients were able to go through the tests that they needed. It's those kinds of things, finding those little windows of opportunity, where you can go in and make a difference.

I spoke a little bit about the nurses I have on staff. The massage therapists also come with a conventional background. They're all pretty seasoned individuals; I have one who's a social worker, one who's a nurse but was hired as a massage therapist, one who is actually a psychologist and returned to be a massage therapist, one who's an occupational therapist, and one who's a physical therapist. But they're all massage therapists. They come from a conventional framework, and they incorporate the massage therapy. This was very important for us in our acute care environment, because they understand the medical language.

The acupuncturists are a little different in that they don't necessarily have a conventional background. The one seasoned person we have is a pharmacist on staff who is a Chinese medicine practitioner and is trained in both Eastern and Western herbs. He has helped provide information to physicians at the bedside about those patients who come in with their garbage bags full of things. And he helps to assess for the physician what should and shouldn't be taken at the same time. This also facilitates physician buy-in; it helps them find ways to fill the voids in their education or in their treatment of their patients.

We have a partnership with Northwestern Health Sciences University, which is a chiropractic school that also has traditional medicine and massage. We do 13-week clinical rotations with their students. Part of the reason that I started that partnership was because I could not find practitioners to come into the acute care environment and understand what it is to treat patients who are in medical crisis. It is a very different practice for complementary therapists when they're out in the community versus in a hospital with IVs going on and ventilators and other things. We're creating this acute care experience for these practitioners because our work at Abbott needs to translate to all the other ten hospitals within Allina. That's the vision of the CEO of Allina.

The process is constantly changing. I look at being as integrative and holistic in the process as we are in the delivery of the care. And I put building relationships at the bottom because that truly is the foundation for everything else. We have to create the relationship first before we can actually do whatever it is we want to do. It's sort of just feeling it out, when's the right time to move forward with certain things.

MR. BERRY: Hawaii is a receptive place to do mind/body medicine because of all the Eastern influences. All the cultures bring their own ideas about what constitutes healing practices. The board of directors, from the very start, said they were going to have an integrative medical staff. So, besides having MDs and DOs, they planned to credential other disciplines, other healing traditions, and that includes naturopaths, acupuncturists, chiropractors, healing touch practitioners. We have no Chinese medicine physicians on staff, although there is a credentialing category for that as well. And we also wanted Hawaiian practitioners, but we have no one in that category.

Now, in those categories, we may have one or two people. Why is that? Well, one reason is that we have a small community, so there is not a big pool of practitioners. We don't have 30 or 40 acupuncturists and so forth. The other reason is because they're not used very much. Paying medical staff dues and coming to meetings at first may have sounded like a great idea to practitioners but, eventually, it sort of got to the point where they said, why bother? Nobody's going to call me. We wished that wasn't the case, but that's one of the challenges.

Hawaii has a mandated health plan, so everybody's basically insured, but it doesn't pay for acupuncture and massage therapy and so forth. That is a challenge. And once in a while we can get a grant to pay for some of this, run research projects when we can, but the average patient does not have contact with alternative care providers.

We do have bedside nursing treatment such as massage and healing touch and the Care Channel and aromatherapy and so forth, but in terms of having other healing traditions in the community come in, it's very limited. In some ways, those healing traditions probably work best outside the hospital in longer-term stress-management issues. I tell the physicians that if you have somebody who is obese with diabetes and hypertension, you have 15 minutes to deal with that patient. Why don't you refer the patient to a naturopath who's trained in nutrition and so forth and see if it doesn't help, and that is done from time to time.

Sometimes I feel like we're more bark than we're bite. We have this integrated hospital, and we have all these different healing traditions in the community, but we really don't make it happen every day, and I wish we could.

We do have an integrative healing committee that is populated with physicians and alternative care practitioners, so there's an exchange of information going on, so we continue to try to be our mission.

Interestingly, the Hawaiian practitioners are not involved because there's no way to credential them. Acupuncturists and massage therapists are licensed, but Hawaiian practitioners are not licensed. And as a group, they don't want to be licensed because they come from different traditions, they're trained on an oral basis and there's no way to really test for competencies.

But the Hawaiians came with a very interesting and, I think, a very valuable healing tradition. They use three different ways of treating people. One was called Lomilomi, which is a type of deep massage. From early childhood up through adult, people massaged each other.

Then they have La' Apa' Hou, which was the use of herbs. There are lots of directions about when to pick an herb, what season, what time of day, and so forth, and how to use the herb. Some of that is still used a little bit, but it's not widely used.

And the third is Ho'o Pono Pono. Ho'o Pono Pono means to make right. I thought this was probably the most fascinating thing about the Hawaiian culture. If you had a disease, it was felt that you were probably angry with somebody, and you needed to sit down and talk about it—almost like an encounter session. I see that happening around our community and in the hospital every so often when the families come together, particularly when there's a drug addiction, and they'll use Ho'o Pono Pono to sort of make the person own up to their issues. The Hawaiians have a tradition after you do this of eating and then washing in the ocean.

Anyway, I guess I'd go back to say that we wish we would do more, and we're really trying to do more. But without the referral and without the reimbursement, there are just huge challenges to accomplishing that. But I am proud of the fact that our medical staff does welcome and does actually credential a wide range of people.

MS. CUOCO: I had a question for Stan. It sounds like your environment must be just terrific. Have you thought about creating a center of excellence that can actually draw people from across the country to be there?

MR. BERRY: Actually, we just established the Heart-Brain Center at North Hawaii Community Hospital. Earl Bakken believed that there is a strong connection between the heart and the brain. Most Americans are succumbing to cardiovascular diseases, strokes, and heart attacks, and our population actually has a higher incidence of those kinds of disease processes. So we're looking at addressing all the issues from where you live in the community and the groups you associate with, how do we teach you to recognize symptoms or change your diet, what can we do from a technology standpoint, and so forth. So, we hope we become a center for excellence so that people on the island will come to our hospital for basic cardiovascular care because we have a competency in that, and then that will generate some income to fund other things. We can build on that strength and hopefully do more in the area of diabetic wellness.

We've always had an idea of attracting people from around the world and certainly across the states. We just haven't got them there yet. One advantage we have is this coastline that's full of resorts and where big homes are being built. People realize that if they have a heart attack, they're pretty well restricted to recovery care on the island, so we're able to turn that concern into pragmatic giving to the hospital.

MS. MITCHELL: Nancy had mentioned about the pharmacist. There are some real challenges and some positive changes that are going on related to integrative medicine tied to the pharmacist on the patient care unit. Hospitalized patients usually don't know that there's a pharmacist in the hospital. Hopefully, that's changing with pharmacists being active in the patient care on the unit, doing clinical profiles, looking at the patient's home medication at the time of admission or shortly thereafter, and reviewing physician orders.

There are significant quality improvement opportunities if you can get the pharmacist closer to the care of the patient, and you can add some complementary therapies if you involve them in the care of the patient.

MS. VANMEETREN: We have decentralized, and we have clinical pharmacists on the floors, and they now speak to the physicians. They do the rounding with physicians. We've been able to make great strides in more appropriate use of expensive drugs. They easily justify themselves based on cost. Within six months, the cost savings contributions by a clinical pharmacist on the unit interacting with the patients and the physicians and the staff are significant.

MS. MOORE: One of the things that the Joint Commission now requires as a patient safety goal is medication reconciliation. Look at how many people have readmissions, get really sick, because that hasn't been happening. They have duplicate medications, and they have medications that interact with one another, and one physician doesn't know what another physician ordered.

MS. HENLEY: Our pharmacists are doing the reconciliation. They've been on the units for several years. In Washington, they're looking at prescriptive authority for pharmacists. That would be a pretty significant change. You know, I think that patients are far more likely to tell pharmacists everything that they're using at home—what's in their brown bag—more so than they might with their physicians or even nurses. For us the combination of hospitalists and pharmacists has really made a big difference in terms of spending more time with the patients and having a more coordinated approach.

MS. KNUTSON: Four years ago, we did a survey in all the different admitting areas in the hospital, asking patients what they're taking as far as supplements and herbs, among other things. And if they brought those things with them, we asked if they would discuss this with their physician. We were astounded how many people said, no, I'd give them to my spouse, or my sister's going to bring them in tomorrow so nobody knows. It was more than half of the people that we surveyed.

MR. BERRY: There's faith in what these things are supposed to do. It's amazing. It's almost a blind faith. People sometimes believe in these things more than traditional treatment with science behind it.

MR. FINCH: Who else is doing complementary therapies in their hospitals?

MS. HENLEY: When we became a Planetree affiliate, one of the first things we did many, many years ago was have a conference on Reiki, and our medical staff nearly went over the cliff. They were just beside themselves. So we have taken the stealth approach since then. We just introduce things one at a time and let people get used to them.

One of the things that we did was certify staff members through a very intense course in aromatherapy. They have since gone out and created kits that are available on the units. We have massage therapy. We have relationships with massage therapy schools, so students come in and work with patients if they're interested in that.

We just opened a new cancer center, and as part of that we developed a wellness center in conjunction with a naturopathic university in Seattle. That has made a big difference. We're kind of going with some of the more mainstream things, but we also have a culturally diverse population. So we're open to a lot of things so long as they don't do any harm.

MS. KNUTSON: Well, our biggest, our most difficult challenge was talking about energy work, and now it's part of the electronic medical record. The language is actually in there. So we have flow sheets on Meridien assessments and touch. We found a couple of physicians that actually were doing energy work and not telling people.

MS. HENLEY: We had one of ours who was actually a Reiki practitioner. Nobody knew it until probably about three or four years ago.

MS. MOORE: We have an advisory group of physicians from different specialties, acupuncturists, spiritual care, nutritionists, administration, and some other folks, that guide what we do in the hospital. Acupuncture was a big one for the medical staff. I think it was primarily about not really understanding it and not feeling competent themselves to be able to credential something they were not familiar with. So what we did was to utilize our human resource process and have an accupuncturist on call the same way you would have an on-call nurse or any other on-call person. It's not widely used though. Again, there is a cost issue for the patients—it's offered to the patients, but they may not choose it because they're told it may be something that they have to pay for themselves. It may not be covered by their insurance.

The other area we're looking at using acupuncture in is addressing nausea in postoperative pain. We also offer massage on an out-of-pocket basis for patients and the staff.

One thing I wanted to ask, because I think there's so much opportunity for us to help people, is whether anyone is offering EMDR in your emergency room and other areas. It's an eye movement desensitization therapy.

MS. KNUTSON: We do. We have a psychologist on staff that works with that and then two of our nurses are trained in it.

MS. MOORE: And the response, are you seeing it being very effective?

MS. KNUTSON: It's not a primary therapy that we use. They're pretty clear about when and how they're going to use it, and they usually don't use it alone. None of our therapies are used alone; they're really used integratively. So it's in combination with other things, whether it's energy work or even hypnosis.

MS. CUOCO: Well, we have two things. We have one physician who is an acupuncturist. Actually, he's an anesthesiologist, and he used acupressure before he used acupuncture.

We also have a freestanding oncology center that houses our complementary medicine efforts. We have different practitioners that come in and, again, are paid out of pocket by patients. It's always kind of outpatient driven.

MR. FINCH: So what are the problems with bringing innovative complementary therapies into your hospital?

MR. BERRY: I can talk about the women's center that the hospital operates. We had to employ our OB/GYNs because we were losing them. Reimbursement wasn't enough. So we have four OB/GYNs and three midwives who do most of the primary care. We have one person who's really out there, in terms of believing in blended medicine and wanting to try different things, and others that are very conservative. So you're trying to accept a person's professional opinions about different alternative practices, but there have to be some limits on it, particularly if the hospital is going to employ that person.

MS. CUOCO: I think the biggest limitation is education. The hardest piece is to get people to at least be open enough to learn a little bit about something before they put the walls up. Once you begin to show them that there are outcomes that are positive it opens the door for them to become educated. But that's been a big issue.

MR. FINCH: I think I heard some of you say you're doing things in the area of complementary therapy, but it's not used a lot.

MS. CUOCO: It's not used in the acute side for me right now. It's mainly driven by outpatient needs.

MS. HENLEY: For us it depends on whether it's something our staff members provide or not. So if it's aromatherapy or touch or that kind of thing, it's used frequently. The things that require bringing somebody else in who expects to be paid for the therapy are not used nearly as much.

MS. CUOCO: I would agree. That's really what I mean too, because we do aromatherapy a lot.

MR. BERRY: Same here, 60 percent of our patients get Reiki therapy because the hospital has a full-time nurse and volunteers doing it.

MS. MOORE: I think one of the biggest obstacles is the cultural mind-set that if it's offered by the hospital then it should be covered by my insurance. I think that's probably been one of the biggest barriers.

MS. MITCHELL: I think one of the most significant changes in a care model that has occurred over the last several years in many hospitals across the country was the introduction of the universal care delivery model; it's reducing the transfer of the patient between levels of care. It's called either universal care delivery or acuity-adaptable room. In our experience at Celebration, after six years of implementation the model was changed to include a distinct intensive care unit, with private acuity adaptable rooms otherwise. In a new hospital now being built by Adventist Health System, there will be a distinct ICU based on the Celebration experience. However, there are hospitals across the country that have no distinct ICU. In my experience, it's very hard to do totally universal care at a hospital greater than 60 beds or so.

MS. MOORE: Did Celebration move back to having an ICU because of the need to maintain the competency level of the nurses—what was the reason for moving back?

MS. MITCHELL: The driving force was the ability to recruit and retain critical care nurses when their patient volumes increased and the number of beds increased. And the medical staff really wanted a distinct intensive care unit. While the outcomes and the measures of productivity, quality, and patient and family experience demonstrated the benefits of universal care delivery, the driving force for going back to a distinct intensive care unit was to improve the ability to recruit and retain critical care nurses and to respond to the desires of the medical staff.

MR. FINCH: Let's talk about spiritual care. To get started, Vicky, could you tell us about what you're doing, and then Kathy, could you tell us about your experience at Celebration?

MS. VANMEETREN: I think that identity is really important, and part of our hospital's identity speaks to the spiritual. On the top of our bell tower, we have a cross that stands about 13 feet high. Each of our campuses is named after a saint, and we have a statue of Catherine of Siena holding an olive branch. She has an extended hand, and it's not uncommon for us to see adults or children slide their hand into hers. There's a walkway there and a fountain around the statue, and it's very easy to put your hand there.

We put scripture on the walls. Depending upon where you are in the hospital, there are messages. There's a quote from Mother Teresa, which is "Love in action is service." That is where our own staff actually enter the hospital, so we want to remind them in a subtle way.

There is, in the front lobby, "Love tenderly, walk softly, act justly." And in our maternal-child floor, there's one that always makes me smile that says, "God is eternally pregnant." As you sit in the OR waiting room, there is a scripture that is, "Be still and know that I am God." That's a favorite of mine. I think no matter what happens to people, their anxiety needs to leave them, and so that's what we've tried to do.

We have an ecumenical chapel. You have to meet people where they are. It's not about being Catholic. So we have the Bible, we have the Torah, and we have the Koran. All of those are present and usually laid open in that chapel.

The cross and the mission statement are found in every single department. I feel very strongly that our sisters and that our culture is the thing that resonates with patients. One of our nurses came running down to a sister's office, which is always open. She was appalled because the cross was missing in a room. Whoever was in the room last must have taken it home. Well, the sister smiled and put her arm around her as usual and said, "I would think that they probably need it more than we do." When I ordered the crosses, the sisters ended up ordering a couple hundred. They asked me to put them up with just a little simple nail, so they are very easily taken on and off.

One of the things that our sisters are very protective of is that we have a quiet room on every single floor. It is all about dignity when you have to give those messages, whether they're positive or negative; you need to have a place to go and sit down with people. There are all private rooms in these hospitals, but it is important sometimes to the family to be able to ask questions away from the patient.

MS. MITCHELL: When you visit any Adventist Health institution in the United States or in the world, you'll hear some commonality that relates to whole-person health, because it's who we are. One of the ways that we communicate that to other people is eight principles of healthy living. Is this about spirituality? In some ways it is, and in a lot of ways it's not. A lot of this is transferable and has nothing to do with spirituality. On the other hand, it all has to do with spirituality.

An important thing that's going on within Adventist Health is the presence of spiritual ambassadors. These are employees who are more comfortable than others with spirituality and recognizing spirituality and maybe even spontaneous prayer. We introduce new employees to this spiritual ambassador program at the time they are hired. They're offered the opportunity to become a spiritual ambassador. There is in-service training for spiritual ambassadors. Fellow employees who are not spiritual ambassadors know who the spiritual ambassadors are, so they can call upon them not only for patients and family members who might be in need but for one another. They can seek them out in times of need. They're recognized annually when there are hospital functions. If there's a picnic or similar event, they even have T-shirts that recognize them as spiritual ambassadors. There are times throughout the year when you have opportunities to celebrate patient care experiences and testimonies of your patients and families, and there's nobody better to tell those stories than the spiritual ambassadors. They are great folks, and they certainly impact patient satisfaction, patient loyalty, and staff retention. They're part of our spiritual program.

MR. FINCH: We've heard presentations from two hospitals where spirituality plays a major role. Tell me how spirituality is addressed in the other hospitals.

MS. CUOCO: Everyone has some religious background, and we try to make it so there is acceptance of spirituality. We don't have crosses up or Bibles in the room, but there is a sense of spirituality throughout the whole organization that is related to caring for another human being. And, you know, it sounds very religious, but laying hands on is what we all do. From the person who parks your car to the person who actually escorts you into the MRI or into the OR, people believe that what they're doing is, in some form or fashion, in the spirit of caring and healing.

MS. HENLEY: We emphasize spirituality in our orientation as we talk about our standards of performance. We talk about the fact that ours is a sacred trust, that it's not denomination specific but still we have a sacred trust. And we do several things, I think, that help to emphasize that. We do a blessing of the hands for our caregivers, so that's something that really grounds them. In our cancer center, when someone is done with their chemotherapy, there's a ceremony and the staff sing. They all come together and sing as someone leaves them, regardless of what the prognosis is. It's something that the staff developed. And then, for home health and hospice, we do an annual memorial service and invite the families of hospice patients who have died to come back and have a time of remembrance using some of the various symbols of letting go—candles and smoke and things. Again, this is totally developed by our staff and put into place by them. One of our facility redesign elements was taking a patient room and creating kind of a quiet-room chapel that is nondenominational. Every major religion is represented in banners that go around the room.

MS. KNUTSON: It was interesting that when we first began to use the language of "mind, body, spirit," our chaplain office said, "Wait a second, we're spirit." There was a little bit of territorial concern about this. We discussed with them what we meant by that language, and they changed the department name from chaplaincy to spiritual care.

We also worked with our facilities people regarding the native healers that come into the hospital. We have a big Native American population and large Hmong, Tibetan, and Somali populations. So we worked through some of the politics of being able to bring in native healers and spiritual guides, working with our facilities people to shut off the sprinklers when they wanted to do smoke or similar things.

MR. FINCH: How do you talk about spirituality in a secular organization? How do you talk about it in terms of the business of the hospital?

MS. CUOCO: I think it's a spirit of healing that is the mission. We have a strong religious aspect in our pastoral care, and pretty much all of our local ministries are part of our hospital. So it's in that way that religion is promoted.

We're healers, that's who we are in the organization. There is a mind-set that is different. The people who have embraced the concept of healing as we do, in the sense of mind/body/spirit, whether they are physicians, or nurses, or our housekeeping people, they can talk about the concept of healing easily.

But for another faction, it's just a business. There are two different camps. But we speak about being healed freely, and if people are uncomfortable, we just move forward with it. I think there's probably a critical mass who are in their vocation for spirituality and healing, in comparison to people who are not.

MS. KNUTSON: We speak more about what gives purpose and meaning to life, so we don't speak about denomination or religion. When we were developing the medical record forms that our staff use, we included a question about spirituality, but we really ask, "What gives your life purpose, what gives your life meaning?" Sometimes it's about a religion and sometimes it's not, but it opens up a larger discussion.

MS. MOORE: I think for us it was difficult. I think people thought that spirituality was religion. Spirituality may manifest itself through one's religious beliefs, but it really is about who we are and how we work together. It's purpose and meaning in work and service to others. It took dialog, it took discussion, it took people being able to talk about their discomfort with the word "spirituality" and how they personally defined it.

MS. VANMEETREN: In opening a new hospital, I was interviewed by many reporters who wanted to do a piece on it. Typically, they asked how the hospital is different than any other hospital. And I tried to say that we are like no other secular hospital in that we address body, mind, and spirit. I really think that it's not about religion as much as it's about paying attention and listening to the spirit of a person.

MR. FINCH: Grace, would you talk about physical environment and its relationship to healing?

MS. HENLEY: We have had the opportunity to design some new facilities. We have very old facilities on the main campus, where we do our acute care. The facilities range from a building that was built in 1958 to a building that just opened last year. At our specialty campus, the facility started out as a TB sanitarian and has been kind of pieced together.

As we have done our designs, we've been fortunate to be able to use the same architect for several years. He has actually been to Planetree conferences with us, and we've sent him on tours of other Planetree facilities. As we've designed our new facilities, we've tried to coordinate the look. In our family childbirth center, there is a totally separate entrance for women coming in for childbirth. They have their own parking areas, available to family members as well.

The next building we were able to build was our cancer center, which also features integrated, open, inviting, very northwest architecture. We wanted no barriers in our buildings, so we use community-type nurse's stations. There are benches, table tops and chart review places right outside the rooms. The nurse's station is a very low desk, with no barriers. It's a gathering place. We have a lot of our family conferences in this seating area. So it's not unusual to walk by and just see families sitting there taking a break. Patient charting and all of the physician charting happens at the low desk in an open area.

In our design, we have tried to bring the outside in. We live in a beautiful area in the Pacific Northwest, and so we have a lot of big windows. In our cancer center, the chemotherapy bays have floor-to-ceiling windows.

Each of our newer units has an active family area and a quiet family area, and they really are pretty spectacular. The active family areas have kitchens and play areas for the children. We have all kinds of little toys and things for kids. For many years we have used aquariums in different places. It's part of Seattle and the water, and so we have them in various places.

We use stained glass and have discovered that this is a great opportunity for benefactors. People like to donate things like that.

We have tried to incorporate healing gardens throughout all of our facilities. They are spaces that everyone takes some time to go through. We have physicians whose offices are just to the west of our building, and they will always make a point of walking through the healing garden to get into the facility. And every one of our healing gardens has a water feature for the sound and the serenity that comes with it.

MS. VANMEETREN: Well, physical design has kind of been my life. When I came to Catholic Healthcare West, they had one of the oldest hospitals in town. They decided that Henderson was the fastest growing city in the United States at that point, and they would build. The result is the Siena Campus, which was built six years ago.

I think the key advice is to get a professional architect who knows you and knows how to design hospitals. They allowed us to design from the ground floor, and we included our staff, our physicians, and our community in the design. One of the things that we did was ask the question, "What is a healing environment to you?" I tried to get input from every imaginable type of worker, community member, family member, and physician. They all had different perceptions of what that is, and so we tried to address them.

The other thing I would say is that, absolutely, ask your own staff, because they come up with some of the most fabulous ideas. When we were building our campus, right before we opened, we did a mock exercise. We put volunteers on the gurneys. It was really for IT. We sent them around to make sure that there was connectivity with the network. Six years ago we were so excited that we were going to have computers everywhere. So here we are down at admitting, and as you walk in the front door, here's a big admitting section. Our IT manager was bragging about these expensive computer carts. One of our clerical people said, "Well, if we have these expensive carts, then what are we doing sitting down here. Just let them go up and get in their jammies and then we'll come up and admit them." I remember, because I was standing there at that moment, that everybody just kind of stopped like that was such an obvious, good idea. And I will tell you that within two months it worked out. The thought is we are never going to refuse anyone for any kind of care, so we greet patients, take them straight up, let them get in their jammies, and then a couple of hours later send someone up. It makes our customer much happier. In our new facility, the admitting department is not in the front of the hospital. So that was a design that was just a fabulous idea.

We have no paging, a quiet atmosphere. Certainly, we believe art is a part of healing and we have some major donors in this facility that have given some great art. Private spaces, scripture and sayings, and then cleanliness. You need to see that it's clean, and there should be no hospital smell. I don't know how to describe it other than we think it's very important that people don't walk in and say "I hate that hospital smell" when they come in.

MS. MITCHELL: Celebration has a program called "It Just Makes Sense." When new hired employees are in orientation, they are shown a video about how environmental care is everyone's responsibility. Everyone picks up trash; everyone tidies up areas. Hospitals get challenged with maintaining the environment unless everybody takes care of it. And trying to get capital allocation for restoration is challenging. Celebration today, nine years later, really does look like it did the day the doors opened. One of the reasons for that is we have a system in place to maintain the environment.

MR. BERRY: I think what we're saying is you have to major in the minors, all the little stuff. I mean, we constantly battle employees who want to stick stuff up on the walls, make paper signs or keep a public area like an admitting office cluttered up. Maybe their home is cluttered and so now their workspace is cluttered, and we have to stay on them about it.

MS. HENLEY: We have dollars available for things that need doing. When I go out on rounds I say, "Is there anything you need?"

And they say, you know what, something ran into the wall over there and it really needs to be repaired. We have dollars available to address this quickly. It's the same thing, if we need new blood pressure cuffs. It really helps with people catching things ahead of time before they get really big.

MR. FINCH: Abbott Northwestern had an established hospital and added a new section to it.

MS. KNUTSON: Yes, we try to get away from calling it the old and the new. Philanthropic dollars are what really helped to make it happen. We hired an architect who is very "green" oriented. He took that concept and the five elements of feng shui and created a pretty magnificent building. We involved people in the community whenever we could. And now we're looking at all our housekeeping supply components—what kind of chemicals we're using—and moving into more green products. With the challenge of finding capital, I think you have to go to philanthropy these days. We're just trying to maintain the normal things with the budget that we have. In the outpatient center that we developed two years ago, the Institute for Health and Healing, we just added four more treatment rooms. We actually put in a bamboo carpet that has a little foam piece underneath that does not hold any kind of bacteria. It's looking outside of what the normal products are that a hospital uses. Our architect basically travels the world looking for the best products. And he gets to do that because we have a couple of donors who want to get him out there to get the best things.

MR. BERRY: Our hospital opened in 1996. The community really wanted it to be different from traditional hospitals. It was designed from the ground up to be a special place.

The whole hospital is really a healing environment. We have the advantage of being small, so there are no elevators, and we have skylights. All of the rooms are private. All of the surgery rooms have glass slider doors that open onto gardens, either internal gardens or external gardens. We can open up and enjoy that fresh mountain air.

Earl Bakken was very influential in designing the hospital. Earl is the founder of Medtronic, the biomedical company based in Minneapolis. He came to Hawaii and decided to retire there but then couldn't stay retired, so he got involved with this hospital project. He really had a lot of influence in convincing people that ideas about integrative care ought to be built into the hospital. So, with the music, gardens, and artwork, the building itself is a healing vessel.

CHAPTER 11

Measuring and Sustaining Success

This chapter continues the discussion among roundtable participants that began in Chapter 10, with a shift in focus. In this phase of the discussion, the participants were asked to reflect on what they believed to be the most significant issues in sustaining the changes they described in Chapter 10. They were asked in particular about their personal approaches to leading change in their organizations and how they made a case within their organizations for the innovations they advocated. As in Chapter 10, Michael Finch, Ph.D., facilitated the discussion. In this chapter, he was joined by Wayne Jonas, M.D., director, the Samueli Institute, and Christine Choate, Ph.D., deputy director, Samueli Institute, who also engaged in the discussion. The following individuals from seven study hospitals participated in the roundtable, and their conversation has been edited for this chapter:

Stan Berry, president and CEO, North Hawaii Community Hospital

Christine Choate, deputy director, Samueli Institute

Linda Cuoco, vice president, Patient Care Services, and CNO, The Valley Hospital

Mike Finch, senior fellow and consultant, Optimal Healing Environments, Samueli Institute

Grace Henley, assistant administrator, Human Resources, Highline Medical Center

Wayne Jonas, director, Samueli Institute

Lori Knutson, director, Institute for Health and Healing,
Abbot Northwestern Hospital

Kathy Mitchell, CNO, Adventist Bolingbrook Medical Center

Nancy Moore, vice president, Healing Health Services, and
CNO, St. Charles Medical Center

Vicki VanMeetren, president, St. Rose Dominican
Hospitals–San Martín Campus

MR. FINCH: When we think about building healing environments in hospitals, how do you define success? How do you measure it?

MS. VANMEETREN: One of the measures I think is when the medical staff, which is a major partner in your community, wants to come there, wants to be there, wants to be a part of the organization, and wants to be on the committees. I think that's a success, when they clearly see you're set apart from the others.

MR. BERRY: Physicians have a sense of pride in our hospital, and I think that's what you're saying, too. They want to be connected to a successful hospital where their patients give them good feedback. There are a lot of urban areas where physicians have a lot of choices, so you've got to be different.

MS. CUOCO: I think, besides physicians, it's a recruitment tool for our staff. When you talk about nurses or any of the clinical professions right now, there's a shortage everywhere. But we don't have a problem with recruiting. And it's partly because it's a beautiful facility and when people come in, they feel good about where they work. It's more part of the culture and wanting to belong to a winning team.

My turnover rate has gone down, but not as much as I'd like. Last year we ended at 9.5 percent. We probably saved well over $3.4 million in decreasing our turnover, and we also eliminated agency. And then we created and launched the dream, which is the Center for Advancement of Holistic Knowledge and Practice. We've just been asked by the New York Presbyterian Association Group, with 22 hospitals, to start consulting to see what portions of this can be implemented there.

MS. KNUTSON: It's the retention piece too for us. And, obviously, it's patient outcomes. If you show that you've improved patient outcomes, hopefully this leads to improved financial outcomes.

MR. FINCH: Any outcomes in particular? What do you look at for outcomes?

MS. VANMEETREN: You can't say that one outcome measure is necessarily more important than the other. So I think that we take the obvious ones that are measured by outside parties, whether it's regulatory or nonregulatory. Then we add our own internal measures.

MR. BERRY: I think it's hard to measure success objectively. It goes back to what somebody said—do the right thing for your patients. That's a mission-driven, subjective outcome. If the patients are happy, they want to come back to your hospital. But it's hard to measure.

MS. MITCHELL: I think the easiest one is it clearly affects recruitment and retention. And it's really easy to see how recruitment and retention affects clinical outcome. I think anybody can put their arms around that.

MS. MOORE: Patient satisfaction. I know—to echo what people are saying—that outcomes are so multidimensional. It's really hard to pull one thing out. But if our patients feel good and they want to come back, and nurses want to stay and doctors want to bring their patients and they feel good about working in the environment, to me that's it.

One patient told me a story. She had told her nurse this is really a beautiful hospital. And the nurse said, "It's beautiful on the inside, too." That's it. That's what we're looking for.

MR. FINCH: One of the things that we hear from everybody in one form or another is, "We do this because it's the right thing to do." If I hired you to consult with me in my hospital, I might agree that it's the right thing to do, but what are the other things that go into the thinking?

MS. MOORE: I think you have to translate it into that internal investment formula. The replacement of a nurse is about $60,000, and that really helps.

MR. FINCH: What are two or three of the most important lessons you've learned doing this work that you've done?

MS. KNUTSON: Patience, tolerance.

MR. BERRY: I think you have to let these things creep into the organization. You just can't go to the medical staff and lay out a healing-touch program.

MS. CUOCO: And listening. Because if you don't listen—I mean as a leader you push these things out there. But you have to listen to see if your organization, your staff, are ready. And if you listen well, you know when they're ready for a big surge of something, and when you need to hold back and let it just organically grow.

When I think of the leadership qualities that make it happen, we have a phrase at St. Charles, we call them monomaniacs. They have a passion for something. With every successful initiative that we have, there's been a monomaniac behind it, somebody that was on fire making it happen, and they never give up. They keep going for it. They run into obstacles, and they find a way around them, or they're quiet for a while and then they bring it back the next time.

Eventually, it has to have physician support. And I think in the hospital setting sometimes you don't start there because, especially, alternative therapies have been pretty threatening to the medical staff historically. I think we're getting through some of that now, but eventually you need the physician champion working with that hospital-based champion to move things forward.

MS. MITCHELL: I think primarily across our company it's maybe called different things, but holding people accountable to some type of a plan like you have for other aspects of your business, that you have a written plan, you know very specifically what your intentions are, and then how outcomes will be measured, and then, have you done it or haven't you? What are your measures, and where are you at? Are you doing these things or aren't you? And how are you improving? From department to department across the hospital, it's expecting some deliverables that relate to aspects of care that are important and set us apart from the competition. Because we feel as though this is what makes us different and is important to the care of patients.

MR. FINCH: How about operational issues? Any advice?

MS. HENLEY: Yes, slow and stealthy. One of the things I think that we're coming to grips with is that you can create the environment, you can have the intention, but if you have a single "problem child" in any area, it will negate everything you've tried to do. You can teach a lot of things but you can't teach nice. We've actually asked our managers to classify their staff as low, medium, or high performers. They use the high performers as mentors, move the medium people up or out, and call me to deal with the low performers. It's made an enormous difference.

MR. BERRY: I think you can create healing environments with the gardens and the facilities and your staff, but I've given up a long time ago thinking we're not meeting the mission if we don't have acupuncture showing up every day because I can't solve the reimbursement issue. So you have to separate that in your mind. Because you don't have complementary care providers patrolling the hospital doesn't mean you're not accomplishing a healing environment.

MS. MOORE: I think that's so true. It's not the program, it's not the activity—it's the consciousness of the people. It's the ongoing focus on the growth and development of the consciousness of the organization. I was really struck by the pacing comment. How much change can people accommodate? Being able to judge that. Because there have been times where we've been too slow and times when we've been too fast, where it was too much, and people just kind of fuzzed out and couldn't accommodate it.

You have to keep watching for how well things are working. We've had an organization structure that worked really well for us, and we were doing really well. We had good outcomes, but we stayed with that structure too long because it was comfortable. By the time we realized it, we had lost ground, and it was hard to get back. And there's a certain amount of humility in never thinking you're there; there's always more.

MS. VANMEETREN: I think as a leader you have to learn to be a change agent. You have to show by example. If you don't show by example, it won't happen.

MS. MOORE: One other thing I think is important is courage. I think we've hung on to people who really weren't staying engaged and moving forward, and that ends up hurting a lot of people. If they're in a management position, everybody under them and the people working with them are affected as well. I had a person tell me recently that he equated courage with leadership. That really resonated with me.

MS. KNUTSON: I think there's the need to do a lot of check in. I'm always asking what people need or what their thoughts are, engaging them in dialog, not just waiting for people to come and tell you what's not going right.

MS. MITCHELL: In the new hospital, I really want to try to do a better job of meeting the needs of the physicians. How do we do a better job of communicating with physicians? It is really challenging. The physicians did see readily the benefits to them of universal care delivery. They were not being called at all hours of the day and night to move patients to accommodate the next admission. The calls stopped because the patient was not being moved. Physicians were not being called to rewrite orders, but they still want the intensive care unit.

MR. FINCH: Leaders come and go. I hate to say that to all of you, but you know that's true. So, how do you sustain something like this? Or, what are the threats to sustaining these efforts?

MS. HENLEY: You know, we're actually on the opposite side of that. We have eight people in executive positions, and our average tenure is almost 20 years with those eight people. Two of them have been with us less than seven years. We really have had to look for people in our organization who are champions of what we do and the enthusiasm really gets carried forward.

MS. MOORE: In a hospital, if the CEO doesn't adopt the philosophy of the previous CEO, the philosophy will change because the new CEO will set the standard. You have to educate the board so it understands the healing environment—why it's important, all the things we talked about. But the board turns over too, so there's a part of it that really is impermanent. I think probably the best thing is to do all those things: educate your board but really set up a deep foundation in the organization, in the culture, in the consciousness of the organization, and accept that it's not going to always be the same.

MS. VANMEETREN: I don't think it should be the same.

MS. CUOCO: I think leadership can come and go, but if the front line embraces the idea of the healing environment, all of the practices that go around it will continue. I don't think it's as much at the top level as I do at the level that's hands on with the patient.

MS. KNUTSON: I would agree with you 100 percent.

MS. MITCHELL: There will be changes or improvements in the healing environment. In the leadership change that occurred at

Celebration Health, there were significant changes in the nursing model. And usually when you have a change in a significant position in leadership in an organization, it's not just one person. You'll see multiple changes that occur later. But in our case, the healing environment remained. Significant changes occurred in relationship to nursing and the nursing model and care delivery but not in the healing environment.

MR. JONAS: I have a question as to what the role of some of the more hard outcomes is. In terms of the evidence for particular programs actually having an impact, is there a business case?

MS. KNUTSON: We started out by doing a small pilot study working with a few of the DRGs that were the most costly for the organization. One of those was hip fractures. We looked at an integrated approach, not one single modality, because that's not our practice. We looked at pharmaceuticals, the pain management side of it, which is typically the thing that keeps people in the hospital the longest. That is not only because of the pain but because of the narcotics and all the subsequent things that happen from that. We only had 11 patients in our study, but we showed a $2,000 savings. The orthopedic physicians were the toughest group for us to even nudge our way in the door. When we were able to show our results, the referrals from them increased dramatically.

MS. MITCHELL: You've probably heard about the seaside imaging environment at Celebration. It's very much a beach feeling. We used the seaside because whether you're a little person or an elder, everybody loves the beach. It's a surprise to people. It's very beautiful, very healing. There are smells like suntan lotion, and the beach, the sounds of seagulls and the seashore, and you walk on a boardwalk. There are cabanas—it's the seaside. We have had a lower incidence of cancellation since doing this, and lower utilization of pain medication and anesthesia, so there is a cost savings resulting from creating that healing environment.

MS. CUOCO: I think it's extremely important, no matter what you do, to have measurable outcomes that, across the board, people will understand. It's one thing to talk about intuitiveness and healing and all of that, but the bottom line is, if you're going to add on two, let's say, nurse practitioners, what's the outcome? We measure very simple things like patient satisfaction, turnover, recruitment, medication errors, and falls. If the hospital does well in these comparisons, you begin to ask why. And sooner or later you get to the nugget of a healing environment. We talk about our ratios, we talk about our preparation of our staff, we talk about falls, we talk about falls with injuries. But there are very few global databases that you can use to compare those outcomes. There isn't anything that drills down to that level at this point.

The last piece is aromatherapy. We're actually doing research right now with lavender and how it reduces use of a specific drug for elderly patients. We found that this drug has bad effects for elderly patients, like falls and sleepwalking, so we started experimenting with lavender. Two or three drops of lavender are placed on a 2 X 2 card on the side of a bed. We're doing studies now that show reduced use of sleep medications, and we've also reduced our falls by a great deal. And for each one of our falls, we've estimated it's about $150,000 of added cost, even if liability issues are not raised. We've been able to reduce our liability. Not that we can say lavender did it, but it is one of a multitude of things that we were able to do that decreased the use of drugs on patients at night.

MS. VANMEETREN: We have talked about measuring success. Success is generated by creating the environment that people want to work in and patients want to go to.

MS. KNUTSON: The luxury, at least in our case, is that we were given a time frame in which we could create the infrastructure to have this healing environment and get the right people to do the right work and create the right partnerships. We were allowed that. We didn't need to have proof ahead of time in order to make it happen. We were given the luxury of making it happen, and now we have to provide the proof that it should stay around and we should keep doing it. So we're at that place where now we've got the infrastructure, we've been collecting the data, and now we need to build the case.

As far as administrative support, I've been with the organization for 22 years. Administration changes more often than the bedside practitioners. So it's constantly having the right dialog at the right time with the right person. And I think again it goes back to a little bit of intuition, knowing where you need to be and how you navigate with administrators at the right time. The bottom line, in our case, is to speak about money. How does this impact length of stay; how does this impact patient satisfaction; how does it impact the view of the outside community of who we are, because that's what's going to draw our patients; and how does it impact our relationship with physicians. We employ some physicians, but we have independent practitioners who refer to the hospital. Whenever I present to the board about a new practice model that I want, I always have a pro forma available so that I can show some possible financial outcomes. We also have a lot of experiential opportunities for administration, physicians, nurses, and other groups, including philanthropists, that we've brought on board.

The creating of the culture is in all of these elements. It's really being a part of every opportunity. Right now, I'm on 17 different hospital-wide committees. I chair 5 of the 17. It's about being visible, and it's about being out there. Now that it's becoming more of the fabric of the organization, I'm beginning to withdraw from some of these committees, because it's a little much. But all of my nurses are on hospital-wide nursing committees. We position ourselves everywhere we possibly can throughout the organization so that the voice for holistic care is constantly part of the discussion. I think that has been key for our organization, just to be visible and for it to be known as part of the fabric of who we are. There's something in you that's driven to do this.

MR. JONAS: Is there pressure for this proof?

MS. CUOCO: I think there's pressure, but I think, depending on the leadership that dictates it, whether it's the president or the board, it's incumbent upon all of us as change agents and leaders to not wait for them to come and ask us. We need to show them the results so they don't have to ask the question. Before I spend money, I say, "this is what

I project, this is what we'd like to do, this is what I think is an outcome, and I'll report back to you 60, 90 days from now." So I'm proactive.

MS. KNUTSON: That is important, constantly feeding hospital leaders and the board with information. I think this is really important.

MS. CUOCO: I think leadership is an instigator at times, but for sustainability I think it needs to be organic and the staff has to embrace it. But I don't think it will ever remain the same. I think what we started at Valley is already different from the original dream, and it's turned out better. I want the generation that follows to take what we've learned, capitalize on it, and move it out even farther.

People don't understand a healing environment, but they do understand when they walk into the organization they feel safe, they feel welcomed, they feel cared for, and if they have a problem, they are going to be told about it.

MS. CHOATE: Each of you believes strongly that this is a model for your hospital. To what extent do you dream that this is a model that will be created across the country as far as the delivery of healthcare? And what are the barriers to that happening? And what are some of the things that you see happening that can really facilitate this?

MS. HENLEY: One of the barriers that I think we've seen is a lack of imagination. If you can't imagine that your facility can be different because it's older, that's a real constraint. We've been pleased that we've been able to do some of the things we've done with older facilities just through imagination and staff. Lack of imagination, I think, is a real barrier.

MS. KNUTSON: I would agree. I think in the healthcare world we look at scarcity. We tend to focus on scarcity. And I think we should start focusing on abundance. It really is just a frame of mind. Abundance is not just in dollars but in the creativeness of individuals that work with us. When I look at some of the opportunities that we've had with people within our organization, there's abundance out there, and we just have to look at it that way instead of focusing on scarcity.

MS. MOORE: I think one of the concerns is we're all acute care settings. The real work that needs to happen is how to empower people. We're culturally so dependent on the doctor to tell us what to do. What are those models that really shift our culture to more personal ownership of health? And then, also, that spiritual component of grace in old age, life-death transition that is not based on fear.

MR. BERRY: These things all bring a competitive edge to our institutions. I think to the fact that we can differentiate our hospital and have more physician support and more patients, it provides a competitive reward. Now, I think everyone's going to move in that direction. That's just the way it is. So we've got to find the next generation, the next level to move to, and others can't do it because they don't have the capital or the imagination or have other constraints.

I don't think reimbursement is the issue, although reimbursement drives capital. For our hospital, we can never make it on reimbursement. We lose on operations, but the community supports us because it really likes what we're doing. It's a combination of not only high touch but also the high tech, because you have to have both. You can't be one or the other, because it's not a complete picture.

MS. KNUTSON: I want to comment on the whole reimbursement part because, early on, I came to the conclusion that it wasn't going to be about whether we were reimbursed for these services or not. The financial impact had to be around some of the things that Linda discussed, such as nurse retention and decreases in costs. How do you look at this as return on investment? We did a small study with a couple of different DRGs to look at the impact of integrative care practice. We were able to show decreased use of narcotics and decreases in length of stay, and we attached the dollar signs to these changes. Part of my concern with just focusing on the reimbursement is that, as soon as insurance companies see that something will work and decrease costs, then the return is going to be less. So I don't focus just on the reimbursement. It's more philosophically that this is the way we provide care, and how does that help financially in a bigger way.

CHAPTER 12

Lessons Learned

What can hospital leaders learn from the efforts of the eight hospitals described in this book that can help in reinventing the healthcare experience for patients in their own facilities? In this chapter, we address this question using four different areas of focus: vision, motivation, and leadership; strategies for implementation; obstacles to implementation; and challenges to sustainability. We conclude with a brief discussion of factors that we think will shape the future prospects for efforts to reinvent the patient experience.[1]

VISION, LEADERSHIP, AND MOTIVATION

At four hospitals, the building of new facilities or new additions was an important stimulus to rethinking the patient experience in broader terms and was regarded as a key success factor. At two of these facilities (NHCH and ANW), the vision of philanthropists was a major factor in rethinking how to design physical space to enhance the patient and family experience. In some cases, philanthropists also provided support for ongoing programs involving complementary therapies. Respondents in these hospitals expressed a belief that, without the vision and support of these philanthropists, their hospitals would not have attempted to reinvent the patient experience. Two hospitals saw the potential for an enhanced patient experience to create a competitive advantage in attracting patients and attracting and retaining staff. But, interestingly, they did not build marketing campaigns around their efforts, because they were concerned that their communities, including health professionals, might mistakenly assume that the hospital did not provide competitive high-tech, as well as high-touch, care. They did not want to jeopardize the flow of revenues generated by the provision of specialty services. Respondents at all hospitals expressed the opinion that the best way to inform the community of their efforts to reinvent the patient experience was through word-of-mouth opportunities from patients and family members.

IMPLEMENTATION STRATEGIES

The ways in which the study hospitals approached implementation varied, depending on each hospital's capabilities, culture, and leadership. The four strategic components noted in Chapter 1 provide a useful way to organize the discussion of implementation strategies.

Physical Environment

When designing new facilities (three of the hospitals), or new wings and specialty centers (four of the hospitals), all sought to create a physical environment that would enhance the patient experience and support the healing process. Hospital leaders believed that this emphasis also facilitated fund-raising and enhanced their ability to attract and retain nurses and members of the medical staff. In this way, it supported the implementation of other components of their strategy. They also believed that a carefully designed physical environment could facilitate the healing process for patients and that, at present, most hospital space did not do this effectively.

Nursing Practice

The development of a new approach to nursing care received particular emphasis at three hospitals. These hospitals reported that their attempts to redefine the therapeutic role of nurses in caring for patients were well received by most nurses. However, some nurses believed that spending more time at the bedside competed with the demands of hospital quality improvement initiatives, especially the installation of electronic medical records systems, and therefore increased job-related stress. This was a minority viewpoint, and nurses who strongly held it typically left to find positions in other hospitals. Their departure actually facilitated implementation, as they were replaced with nurses who were excited by and supported the hospital's new approach to nursing practice.

Complementary Therapies

In comparison with implementing changes in the physical environment and in nursing care, hospital leaders expressed greater concern about introducing complementary therapies in their hospitals. They sought to balance their desire to make these therapies available to inpatients with their concern that this would provoke a negative reaction on the part of medical staff. In general, they took a cautious approach because of this concern. (This issue is discussed in more detail later.)

Spiritual Support

The spiritual aspects of patient care received attention in all eight hospitals. In new construction, it was common for hospitals to include spaces designed specifically for family and patient meditation and spiritual renewal. Two hospitals, both with religious affiliations, established organizational structures to support spiritual aspects of care. Other hospitals pursued a less aggressive implementation strategy, developing spiritual support programs that were not tied to religious practices but were consistent with their particular organizational cultures. In each case, it was assumed that, for some patients, spiritual support could contribute importantly to the healing process.

OVERCOMING OBSTACLES

Leaders in the study hospitals were concerned about how their efforts to reinvent the patient experience would be received by various constituencies, internal and external. They expected to, and in fact did, confront significant obstacles to implementation and used a variety of strategies to overcome them. At WMC, for example, a financial crisis provided an opportunity to implement changes relatively rapidly. Other hospitals took a more measured approach, devoting time and effort to educating groups within the hospital about the changes that were planned, what would be expected of them, and why the changes would benefit patients. In addition, they provided opportunities for experiential learning. For instance, practitioners of complementary therapies made stress-management therapy available to nursing staff, so they could experience the potential benefits of relieving patient stress and anxiety. And in many study hospitals we were told that physicians who initially resisted complementary therapies subsequently became supporters after observing positive effects on patients.

Along with educating nurses and physicians, hospital leadership took care to avoid confrontations with physicians who could organize and solidify resistance to change. Physicians were seen as a powerful constituency in the hospital—a group where "values fit"[2] might be an issue, particularly with respect to offering complementary therapies to inpatients. Consequently, several of the hospitals placed less emphasis on complementary therapies in reinventing the patient experience, while others introduced them gradually, beginning with the least controversial.

Perhaps the most important step that hospital leaders took to address possible implementation obstacles was to emphasize that their hospitals would be both high tech and high touch with respect to patient care. This was important in even the smallest facilities. Maintaining currency in high-tech treatment approaches helped hospital leaders fend off concerns that their efforts to enhance the patient experience signaled an inability, or unwillingness, on their part to compete in the delivery of high-tech specialty services.

SUSTAINABILITY

The sustainability of efforts to reinvent the patient experience depended primarily on the commitment of hospital leadership and secondarily on funding. Most hospital leaders were consistent in their support for these efforts. As a result, reinventing the patient experience became an integral part of their hospital cultures ("It's who we are"). But nursing staff in some hospitals felt that sufficient resources were not being allocated to this goal. To alleviate these concerns, hospital leaders used different means to continuously reinforce the importance of the strategy for patients and the commitment of the hospital to its implementation.

From the standpoint of hospital staff, a change in CEO was a significant threat to their hospital's commitment. This was a relatively frequent occurrence, with two of the eight hospitals having interim CEOs at the time of our data collection visits, and others having replaced their CEOs within the past three years. The fact that the efforts of these hospitals to reinvent the patient experience survived (sometimes multiple) CEO changes suggests that hospital boards selected new CEOs who they believed would support these strategies.

With respect to finances, most hospital leaders felt that their efforts, excluding those involving new construction, likely "paid for themselves." In some cases, fund-raising was relied on to cover program shortfalls or start-up costs for new initiatives. Only twice did hospitals put initiatives in place that were subsequently scaled back or abandoned for financial reasons. Some hospital leaders believed that their strategies contributed to shorter lengths of stay for some patients, reduced use of narcotics, lowered cancellation rates, or reduced infection rates. It is important to note that these views were based largely on anecdotal evidence. There were attempts to measure the impact of specific initiatives on inpatient treatment costs, but the number of patients involved was small, and the findings typically were inconclusive. For the subset of hospitals that emphasized nursing practice, the financial case for sustainability was expressed in terms of reduced staff costs. Nursing leaders in these hospitals believed it was easier to fill nursing vacancies, and nurse turnover was lower, because of their nursing practice approaches and the attractive working environments their hospitals provided for nurses. Given the costs of recruiting and training new nurses,[3] they saw this as convincing evidence that their nursing practice approach reduced costs.

KEY SUCCESS FACTORS

Hospitals were identified as candidates for this study because they had experienced some degree of success in their efforts to reinvent the patient experience. Therefore, in drawing lessons, we cannot compare hospitals that tried, and failed, to reinvent the patient experience, with the study hospitals, all of which succeeded to some degree. Nevertheless, we believe that each case study provides insights into how hospitals in particular environments can implement such strategies and that general lessons can be drawn from the case studies as a group. Three of the most important relate to formulating strategy, garnering support, and managing the change process.

Formulating Strategy

There is no single template for reinventing the patient experience in hospitals.
Reinventing the patient experience does not require changes in public policy, substantial new financial resources, or unique market situations. The study hospitals were able to shape strategies that addressed constraints and take advantage of opportunities that existed in their own environments.[4] For instance, some hospitals found greater support for complementary therapies in their communities than did others. And an emphasis on spirituality was more readily accepted in hospitals that had a religious affiliation or that were located in communities with cultures that embraced spirituality. There is no single strategic "template" for hospital leaders to follow. While this challenges hospital leaders to be creative, it also provides opportunities for hospital staff to be involved in shaping change strategies. That involvement can help secure staff buy-in to the implementation process.

Garnering Support

External pressures and opportunities can be leveraged to garner support for reinventing the patient experience.
Financial challenges drove one community to consider a new vision for its community hospital. In two other cases, philanthropists partnered with hospital leaders to create a vision for a reinvented patient experience. The resources they provided allowed the hospitals to envision changes that would not otherwise have been considered. In two other instances, rapid population growth, or anticipated

growth, in the community was used to support the need for a new hospital, which then incorporated design features that enhanced the patient experience. In general, hospitals can respond in many ways to different environmental pressures and opportunities as they arise. The study hospitals chose to leverage them in support of reinventing the patient experience, even though this carried with it some degree of risk.

Managing the Change Process

Maintaining a clear and consistent focus on benefits for patients is paramount.
Above all, as they managed their ongoing efforts to reinvent the patient experience, hospital leaders repeatedly emphasized to hospital staff and external constituencies that it was the "right thing to do for patients." Keeping a clear focus on this message, and articulating it effectively, was a key to overcoming implementation obstacles in every study hospital. Frequently, hospital leaders asked staff members to reflect on their own hospitalization experiences, or the experiences of family members, as evidence that change was needed.[5]

PROSPECTS FOR THE FUTURE

It is difficult to predict if a significant number of hospitals will commit to reinventing the patient experience and, if so, whether it will be successful. The hospitals described in this book, and hospitals like them, may prove to be anomalies, and may remain so. Relatively little data are available on the number of hospitals that are currently in the process of reinventing the patient experience in a comprehensive way. We believe that the intersection of three factors will determine the future for such efforts: the impact of emerging consumerism in healthcare, the emergence of an evidence base substantial enough to support management decisions, and the ability of hospitals to assess and address patient values.

The Emerging Consumerism in Healthcare

A variety of forces could inhibit future efforts to reinvent the patient experience. For instance, Medicare budget pressures could result in lower payments to hospitals, making it more difficult to sustain nursing models that involve more nursing care at the bedside. Rising interest rates may limit the ability of hospitals to improve patient care environments through new construction or substantial renovations. The need to keep pace with the proliferation of new and expensive diagnostic and treatment technologies could also divert hospital resources and attention away from the sorts of hospital efforts that we have described. In combination, these forces could well result in hospitals that provide technologically sophisticated care, but in a manner and an environment that do not effectively promote healing or recognize diverse patient values.

Other forces are at play that could lead hospitals to evolve in a different direction—one that supports efforts to reinvent the patient experience. Consumers are demanding more information about hospital performance, and the market is responding with comparative reports that include a variety of measures. At this stage, the measures are primarily clinical in nature, but the number of measures addressing the patient experience could expand in the future if consumers find these data valuable. The increasing employer emphasis on high-deductible health plans with greater out-of-pocket costs for consumers means that consumers may face stronger incentives in the future to seek out information on the totality of hospital care, including elements of the patient experience not now reported. This could provide the impetus for more hospitals to undertake innovative efforts to reinvent the patient experience.

Perhaps just as important, healthcare providers—including hospitals—are increasingly being challenged to address limitations in patient function, along with pain, depression, fear, and despair, all of which may be considered components of the way that patients experience illness. Hospitals may be judged in the future, more so than they are now, on their ability to address these dimensions of the patient experience. The hospitals described in this book are attempting to manage the experience of illness for their patients and for patients' families more effectively. They are trying to create more comfortable and patient-friendly surroundings; provide more personalized care and improve interactions and communication with staff; provide treatments focused on healing, including complementary therapies; and offer spiritual support to ease suffering and help patients cope with the profound impact illness can have on identity and purpose in life. In a future healthcare environment where consumers have more significant roles in managing their care, the question is whether these efforts will be effectively communicated to consumers, whether they will be understood, and whether consumers and their primary advisers on medical issues—physicians—will value them when selecting hospitals.

Developing an Evidence Base

A solid evidence base has largely been lacking for many of the programmatic efforts hospitals have undertaken to reinvent the patient experience. The hospitals in this study can be compared with early adopters of organizational innovations more generally. For early adopters, where evidence on which to base decisions is limited, a compelling vision articulated by a trusted leader can be sufficient to motivate organizational change. However, the innovation literature suggests that later organizational adopters typically demand supporting evidence drawn from the experience of early adopters before they will implement an innovation.[6] Numerous studies and reports have pointed to the need for more research in this area.[7] In the existing literature, there are some indications that the physical environment of healthcare, the communication that occurs, the tone and content of medical information provided to patients, and the cultural assumptions that accompany treatment all influence pain, function, well-being, medical utilization, medical errors, and costs.[8] However, this evidence base will need to be strengthened to a point where it can provide clearer guidance to hospital decision makers in the future. This will be a difficult challenge, as outcomes related to spirituality, relationship-centered care, and complementary therapies may not be readily captured by standard measures of clinical processes.[9] For example, current measures of spirituality (one area addressed by hospitals in this book) may not capture the extensive nonreligious character of spiritual experience.[10] Hope and expectancy are other contributors to recovery from illness,[11] yet measures of these concepts are poorly developed.[12] And measuring the true costs of reinventing the patient experience and linking those costs to revenues and patient outcomes in a way that is informative for hospital leaders will also be a challenging task.

Addressing Patient Values

While the rise of consumerism in healthcare could change this situation, to date most efforts to reinvent the patient experience have not come in direct response to consumer demand, but as a reflection of values held by hospital leaders, local philanthropists, and passionate staff. Consumers have played a relatively limited role in the choice of hospital, which has been largely influenced by insurance plan designs and physician preferences. Nor is it clear that their values have influenced the way in which most hospitals organize and deliver care. In fact, it would be accurate to characterize consumers as mostly bystanders in the market for inpatient care to date. To gather the patient's perspective, hospitals are increasingly using surveys, focus groups, and other means. These tools can be useful in evaluating specific aspects of the patient experience, but they are in the early stages of development and use. Hospital leaders could do much more to understand what patients truly value in the patient experience and to incorporate this knowledge in hospital decisions. Especially as the reliance of medicine on sophisticated diagnostic and treatment technologies grows, hospitals will be confronted with increasingly difficult choices in balancing the high-tech and high-touch aspects of care. The technological aspects of medicine can seem impersonal and may be largely invisible to patients, but maintaining currency is critical to attracting medical staff and generating revenues. However, to maintain the trust of their communities and their patients, hospitals will also need to address those experiential aspects of caring and healing that patients value. The future of efforts to reinvent the patient experience will depend to a considerable degree on the willingness and ability of hospital leaders to integrate patient values into their decision-making process.

ENDNOTES

1. We developed these areas of focus by drawing from the general literature on implementation of innovations in organizations (e.g., Rogers, E. 1995. *Diffusion of Innovations*, 4th ed. New York: The Free Press; Klein, K., and J. Sorra. 1996. "The Challenge of Innovation Implementation." *Academy of Management Review* 21 (4): 1055–80; Duck, J. D. 1993. "Managing Change: The Art of Balancing." *Harvard Business Review* 71 (6): 109–18; Kanter, R. M. 1985. "Managing the Human Side of Change." *Management Review* 74 (4): 52–56; Strebel, P. 1996. "Why Do Employees Resist Change?" *Harvard Business Review* 74 (3): 86–92), along with selected literature on innovation in healthcare organizations (e.g., Green, P. L., and P. E. Plsek. 2002. "Coaching and Leadership for the Diffusion of Innovation in Health Care: A Different Type of Multi-Organization Improvement Collaboration." *The Joint Commission Journal on Quality Improvement* 28 (2): 55–71; Weber, V., and M. S. Joshi. 2000. "Effecting and Leading Change in Health Care Organizations." *The Joint Commission Journal on Quality Improvement* 26 (7): 388–99; Garside, P. 1998. "Organisational Context for Quality: Lessons From the Fields of Organisational Development and Change Management," *Quality in Health Care* 7 (Suppl.): S8–S15; Ponte, P. R., G. Conlin, J. B. Conway, S. Grant, C. Medeiros, J. Nies, L. Preskill, and A. Coghlan (eds.). 2003. *Appreciative Enquiry and Evaluation. New Directions for Program Evaluation.* San Francisco: Jossey-Bass).

2. Klein and Sorra (1996).

3. Waldman, J. D., F. Kelly, S. Arora, and H. L. Smith. 2004. "The Shocking Cost of Turnover in Health Care." *Health Care Management Review* 29 (1): 2–7; Geyer, S. 2005. "Hand in Hand: Patient and Employee Satisfaction." *Trustee* 58 (6): 12–14, 19.

4. This is a recognized stage in the implementation of innovations in organizations. Rogers (1995) calls it "redefining" or "restructuring" and says it occurs "when the innovation is re-oriented to accommodate the organization's needs and structure more closely, and when the organization's structure is modified to fit the innovation" (p.394). The innovation, in this case, is broadly conceived to be "reinventing the patient experience" through a set of initiatives intended to enhance the ability of physical space to support healing, redefine nursing roles, introduce complementary therapies, and provide spiritual support in various forms. The study hospitals redefined or restructured these initiatives to "accommodate their needs and structure." Several also changed the hospital structure, creating new units and committees to manage their efforts to reinvent the patient experience.

5. Identifying a "performance gap" can play a critical role in developing support for implementing innovations in organizations. Rogers (1995, 393) defines this as the "difference between how an organization's members perceive its performance, in comparison to what it should be." Leaders in the study hospitals took a unique approach to identifying a performance gap. Rather than relying on data or studies, they appealed to the personal experience of staff members and their families as hospital patients.

6. Rogers (1995).

7. See, for example, Institute of Medicine. 2001. *Crossing the Quality Chasm: A New Health System for the 21st Century.* Washington, DC: National Academies Press; White House Commission on Complementary and Alternative Medicine Policy (WHCCAMP). 2002. *Final Report* March 22; Institute of Medicine. 2005. *Complementary and Alternative Medicine in the United States.* Washington, DC: National Academies Press.

8. Barrett, B., D. Muller, D. Rakel, D. Rabago, L. Marchand, and J. C. Scheder. 2006. "Placebo, Meaning, and Health." *Perspectives in Biology and Medicine* 49 (2): 178–98.

9. Jonas, W. B., M. Schlitz, and M. Krucoff. 2000. "The Science and Spirituality of Healing." Paper presented at the Science and Spirituality of Healing, North Carolina, October 26–29; O'Laoire, S., and W. Jonas. 2003. "Models, Measurement Descriptors and Outcome Measures. In W. Jonas and C. Crawford (eds.), *Healing, Intention and Energy Medicine: Science, Research Methods and Clinical Implications.* New York: Churchill Livingstone, 211–24; Chez, R. A., and W.

B. Jonas. 2005. "Challenges and Opportunities in Achieving Healing." *Journal of Alternative and Complementary Medicine* 11 (Suppl. 1): S3–S6.

10. Koenig, H., M. McCullough, and D. Larson. 2001. "Measurement Tools." In *Handbook of Religion and Health*. New York: Oxford University Press, 495–512.

11. Kirsch, I. (ed.). 1999. *How Expectancies Shape Experience*. Washington, DC: American Psychological Association.

12. Feudtner, C. 2003. "Research Design and Analysis Considerations for Spiritual Care Interventions." *Proceedings: Spiritual Transformation and Health Through the Life Cycle*, 22–41.

Appendix

RESEARCH METHODS

To study the experience of hospitals in implementing consumer-focused innovations, we employed a multiorganizational, case study research design of a type commonly used in comparative organizational analyses over the past three decades (Greene and David 1984; Glaser and Strauss 1965; Weiss and Rein 1970).

Conceptual Framework

Rather than focusing on specific hospital initiatives, we sought to understand how hospitals combined different initiatives into broader strategies. To guide our research approach, we relied on findings from a review of the general literature on implementing innovations in organizations (e.g., Rogers 1995; Klein and Sorra 1996; Duck 1993; Kanter 1985; Strebel 1996), along with selected literature on innovation in healthcare organizations (e.g., Green and Plsek 2002; Weber and Joshi 2000; Garside 1998; Ponte et al. 2003). Based on our review, we identified four areas of focus: the sources of vision, leadership, and motivation for early adoption of consumer-focused innovation; strategies for implementation, especially the factors that influenced choice of components; perceived obstacles to innovation implementation and how they varied with hospital characteristics; and challenges to sustainability. We used these four areas to organize the presentation of our crosscutting study findings in Chapter 12.

Hospital Selection

In selecting hospitals for our study, we sought organizations that had implemented strategies with multiple components. We also sought variation with respect to hospital size, geographic region served, and length of time involved in significant consumer-focused innovation. Hospital selection is discussed in Chapter 1. The experience of our case-study hospitals arguably generalizes to the 200 to 400 hospitals in the United States pursuing similar strategies to reinvent the patient experience, but not necessarily to all hospitals in the United States because, by definition, hospitals voluntarily select to pursue such strategies. This is an inherent limitation in any analysis of early adopters of innovations.

Data Collection

We used a data collection approach that is common in cross-sectional, multiple case study designs, relying on in-person and telephone interviews, media reports, and documentation provided by the hospitals (Weiss and Rein 1970; Greene and David 1984; Firestone and Herriott 1983). We identified potential interview respondents, a priori, by the nature of the position they occupied within the hospital. Separate semi-structured interview protocols were developed for each position (e.g., CEO, CFO, CNO, marketing or public relations executive, chief of the medical staff, initiative champion). In-person interviews were conducted with individuals in these positions as part of site visits carried out from November 2005 through March 2006. In addition, where warranted based on information collected in preparation for the site visit, individuals were added to the list of interviewees (e.g., chaplains, donors, foundation development officers). Three of the authors participated in the collection of interview data and in almost every case at least two authors were engaged in each interview. Both interviewers took notes during the interview, and all in-person interviews were recorded. Due to scheduling conflicts or last-minute schedule changes, four interviews were conducted by telephone. Interviews with between six and ten respondents were conducted in each hospital.

During the visits to the hospitals, a variety of materials were collected that described hospital efforts to implement consumer-focused innovations (e.g., program descriptions, meeting notes, financial information, media releases, organizational newsletters). Hospital websites were used as a source of background data as well. Based on the interview data and these different information sources, we created a detailed case study of each hospital, which then was reviewed for accuracy by key informants. The summary findings presented in Chapter 12 of this book reflect our crosscutting analysis of these case studies.

REFERENCES

Duck, J. D. 1993. "Managing Change: The Art of Balancing." *Harvard Business Review* 71 (6): 109–18.

Firestone, W. A., and R. E. Herriott. 1983. "The Formalization of Qualitative Research. An Adaptation of 'Soft' Science to the Policy World." *Evaluation Review* 7 (4): 437–66.

Garside, P. 1998. "Organisational Context for Quality: Lessons from the Fields of Organisational Development and Change Management." *Quality in Health Care* 7 (Suppl.): S8–S15.

Glaser, B. G., and A. L. Strauss. 1965. "Discovery of Substantive Theory: A Basic Strategy Underlying Qualitative Research." *American Behavioral Scientist* VIII (6): 5–12.

Green, P. L., and P. E. Plsek. 2002. "Coaching and Leadership for the Diffusion of Innovation in Health Care: A Different Type of Multi-Organization Improvement Collaboration." *The Joint Commission Journal on Quality Improvement* 28 (2): 55–71.

Greene D., and J. L. David. 1984. "A Research Design for Generalizing from Multiple Case Studies." *Evaluation and Program Planning* 7 (1): 73–85.

Kanter, R. M. 1985. "Managing the Human Side of Change." *Management Review* 74 (4): 52–56.

Klein, K., and J. Sorra. 1996. "The Challenge of Innovation Implementation." *Academy of Management Review* 21 (4): 1055–80.

Ponte, P. R., G. Conlin, J. B. Conway, S. Grant, C. Medeiros, J. Nies, L. Shulman, P. Branowicki, and K. Conley. 2003. "Making Patient-centered Care Come Alive." *Journal of Nursing Administration* 33 (2): 82–90.

Rogers, E. 1995. *Diffusion of Innovations*, 4th ed. New York: The Free Press.

Strebel, P. 1996. "Why Do Employees Resist Change?" *Harvard Business Review* 74 (3): 86–92.

Weber, V., and M. S. Joshi. 2000. "Effecting and Leading Change in Health Care Organizations." *The Joint Commission Journal on Quality Improvement* 26 (7): 388–99.

Weiss, R. S., and M. Rein. 1970. "The Evaluation of Broad-Aim Programs: Experimental Design, Its Difficulties, and an Alternative." *Administrative Science Quarterly* 15 (1): 97–109.

About the Authors

Jon B. Christianson, Ph.D., holds his doctorate in economics from the University of Wisconsin–Madison and is currently the James A. Hamilton Chair in Health Policy and Management in the School of Public Health, University of Minnesota. His research interests include health insurance, employer initiatives in healthcare, healthcare markets, pay for performance, organizational change in healthcare, and the translation of evidence-based medicine into practice. Professor Christianson has authored or coauthored seven books and more than 150 articles and book chapters. He serves on the editorial boards of several journals, including *Health Affairs* and *Medical Care Research and Review*.

Michael D. Finch, Ph.D., received his degree in sociology from the University of Minnesota. After 14 years on the faculty of the Division of Health Services Research and Policy at the University of Minnesota, he left to become Director of Research Programs for UnitedHealth Group. He is currently a Senior Fellow at the Samueli Institute and a member of the graduate faculty at the University of Minnesota and has appointments in the Carlson School of Management, the School of Public Health, and the Department of Sociology.

Dr. Finch is widely known for his work on the cost, quality, and financing of healthcare in the public and private market and is nationally recognized as an expert in research methods and evaluation. He has received and worked on dozens of federally sponsored grants and contracts, including the Health Care Financing Administration's National Post Acute Care Project, the Second Generation Social HMO Demonstration, the National Institute of Mental Health–funded Youth Development Survey, and the National Institute for Aging–funded Evaluation of the Medicaid Demonstration. His most recent research includes a study on the effects of surgical volume on outcomes in hospitals, an assessment of guideline performance for diabetes, the cost and financing of end-of-life care, and an evaluation of the Hospital Consumer Assessment of Health Providers and Systems (HCAHPS) survey.

Barbara Findlay, R.N., B.S.N., is vice president of the Optimal Healing Environments Program at the Samueli Institute. From 1997 to 2003, she was with the Tzu Chi Institute for Complementary and Alternative Medicine in Vancouver, British Columbia, where she served as coordinator for Clinical Research and Professional Practice and then executive director. Between 2003 and 2005, she held a senior leadership position with the BC NurseLine, a British Columbia Ministry of Health telenursing initiative. This experience provided a valuable opportunity to consider the role of enabling technology in meeting the health needs of Canadians in the context of healthcare reform.

Ms. Findlay's early professional background includes more than 20 years as a staff nurse in a variety of clinical settings, including inner-city emergency departments, and as an educator for patients and health professionals in a community hospital setting. She received her diploma in general nursing (RN) from British Columbia Institute of Technology and her bachelor of science degree in nursing from the University of British Columbia.

A frequent presenter on the issues surrounding integrative healthcare, she has been an active participant in Health Canada's consultation process surrounding integrative healthcare in Canada and has coauthored a number of reports and peer-reviewed articles on this topic.

Wayne B. Jonas, M.D., is president and chief executive officer of the Samueli Institute, a not-for-profit medical research organization supporting the scientific investigation of healing processes and their application in health and disease. He is a widely published scientific investigator, a practicing family physician, and an associate professor at the Uniformed Services University of the Health Sciences. Additionally, Dr. Jonas is a retired lieutenant colonel in the Medical Corps of the United States Army.

Dr. Jonas was the director of the Office of Alternative Medicine at the National Institutes of Health from 1995 to 1998, and prior to that he served as the director of the Medical Research Fellowship at the Walter Reed Army Institute of Research. He is a Fellow of the American Academy of Family Physicians.

In addition to his conventional medical practice, Dr. Jonas has long been interested in various alternative medicine approaches and has conducted research on homeopathy, electroacupuncture, and nutritional supplements. His research has appeared in peer-reviewed journals such as the *Journal of the American Medical Association, Natural Medicine, Journal of Family Practice, Annals of Internal Medicine*, and *The Lancet*. His many book publications include *Mosby's Dictionary of Complementary and Alternative Medicine, Essentials of Complementary and Alternative Medicine* and *The Complete Guide to Clinical Research Methods in Complementary Medicine*. Additionally, Dr. Jonas received the 2003 Pioneer Award from the American Holistic Medical Association, the 2002 Physician Recognition Award of the American Medical Association, and the 2002 Meritorious Activity Prize from the International Society of Life Information Science in Chiba, Japan. His current research interests include projects on Information Biology™, the placebo effect, cancer, biological effects of low-level toxin exposures (hormesis), homeopathy, spiritual and energy healing, and the quality of research outcomes.

Dr. Jonas earned his medical degree from the Wake Forest University School of Medicine in Winston-Salem, North Carolina, and has held leadership positions with a number of organizations and councils such as the World Health Organization, the National Institutes of Health, and the White House Commission for Complementary and Alternative Medicine Policy. He currently serves on the editorial boards of eight peer-reviewed journals and on the advisory or scientific boards of six national and international organizations, including the Susan B. Komen Breast Cancer Foundation and Planetree International.

Christine Goertz Choate, D.C., Ph.D., received her doctorate in health services research, policy, and administration from the University of Minnesota and her doctor of chiropractic degree from Northwestern Health Sciences University. She is currently executive director of the Palmer Center for Chiropractic Research and president of the Choate Group LLC, a research and communication strategies consulting firm. Dr. Choate is also on the faculty at the Uniformed Services University of the Health Sciences. Her professional experience includes tenures as deputy director of the Samueli Institute and as a program official at the National Institutes of Health. She is the author of numerous scientific publications in journals such as the *Journal of the American Medical Association, Annals of Internal Medicine,* and *Controlled Clinical Trials* and is on the editorial board of several peer-reviewed journals. Dr. Choate has served as president of the Bethesda Chapter of the Association for Women in Science and chair of the Chiropractic Health Care Section of the American Public Health Association (APHA). She is a member of the APHA Action Board and the 2006 recipient of the American Chiropractic Association's Researcher of the Year Award.